4.26.78

The O.K. Way to Slim

The O.K. Way to Slim

Weight Control Through Transactional Analysis

Frank T. Laverty

GROVE PRESS, INC./NEW YORK

First Edition 1977
First Printing 1977
ISBN: 0-394-42164-7
Grove Press ISBN: 0-8021-0145-3
Library of Congress Catalog Card Number: 77-5244

Manufactured in the United States of America

Distributed by Random House, Inc., New York

Published by GROVE PRESS, INC., 196 West Houston Street, New York, N.Y. 10014 by arrangement with Prentice-Hall of Canada, Ltd. Published simultaneously in Canada by Prentice-Hall of Canada, Ltd., 1870 Birchmount Road, Scarborough, Ontario, M1P 2J7.

To Joy—

For thirty years of love, growth, and sharing.
It has been yellow roses and sky rockets all the way.

Contents

EXERCISES

ILLUSTRATIONS

Preface

This book is for people who have tried unsuccessfully to lose weight or who are unable to maintain a weight loss. It is for people who are ready and willing to investigate their own situations in order to identify the underlying causes of obesity. People who are concerned about the obese condition of a family member or friend will gain understanding from this material.

For years, I have been haunted by the questions:
- Is obesity a disease of our times caused by inactivity and the abundance of the good life?

or

- Is a person programmed to be fat?

It is my contention that fatness is programmed in early childhood. In the majority of cases, dieters gain back lost weight because they are treating only the symptom—fatness—rather than dealing effectively with the hidden, psychological causes for the disorder.

Overweight people are physically and emotionally ill. Fat fever is our most serious and costly social disease. Unfortunately, there is no magic cure or wonder drug to boil off weight. The only appropriate approach is for sufferers to find out why they have fat fever and then cure the causes and the symptoms once and for all. For fever is cured in the mind not the stomach.

This book prepares a person psychologically for weight control. It does not suggest what a person should or should not eat.

The transactional analysis model for understanding human

behavior is used throughout this book. I have kept away purposely from the more complex transactional analysis theories and defined each concept and term when it is first introduced.

Self-awareness exercises are introduced at appropriate places. A person may complete the exercises as they appear, although it is usually more pleasurable to read through the book first and then complete the exercises at a second reading. For maximum insight the exercises should be completed in the order they appear in the book. The exercises can be done individually, in pairs, or in a group of six or less. Group involvement provides discussion, stimulation, and feedback but it takes much longer to complete the exercises.

This book is not a substitute for therapy. Some disturbed people who are unable to cope with their weight problem alone require professional treatment. However, most people, who are functioning adequately except for the weight albatross, can use these self-awareness exercises without professional assistance. Completing the exercises and reflecting on the contents provide the insights and stimulation for a continuing liberation from fat fever.

Reprogramming is not easy nor is it always comfortable. It means searching the past systematically for keys to behavior and thoughts, learning more appropriate ways to think and behave, and applying the new learning toward a continuing fat fever cure.

I recognize that at times my approaches, descriptions, and terminology differ from those of other authors. I make no excuses for these differences. I use the terminology with which I am most comfortable and suggest applications which are appropriate for use by persons lacking in-depth training in psychology.

I appreciate the interest and understanding of my colleagues Gordon Lippitt and Charlie Stewart who influenced my growth as a behavioral scientist. I am cognizant also that the writings of the members of the International Transactional Analysis Association stimulated many of my thoughts, approaches, and applications. Specifically, I am indebted to Eric Berne for making transactional analysis a public language; to Claude Steiner for his effective writing on scripts and alcoholism which triggered my application to weight control; to Muriel James and Dorothy Jongeward for their example on the self-use of Gestalt experiments; to Thomas Harris, Stephen Karpman, the Schiffs, and the Gouldings for their outstanding inputs to transactional analysis theory; and to the many other authors who shared their thoughts in the *Transactional Analysis Journal.*

I acknowledge the creative and constructive inputs from my wife and business partner, Joy. Her supportive warm strokes made this project a reality.

Management Renewal Limited   FRANK LAVERTY
Ottawa, Canada   November, 1976

CHAPTER
1
Prologue

A nightmare stimulated me to write this book.

In my dream, I was conducting a training workshop. During the session, the participants got fatter and fatter until the room was full of fatty, rancid flesh. I struggled, fought, squeezed, and writhed along the wall until I burst out the door. I woke up standing beside my bed, shaking and gasping for breath.

The nightmare was not a chance occurrence. For months I have been observing the steadily increasing number of noticeably overweight people in my training workshops. In 3 years, the percentage of corpulent participants increased from 22 to 36 percent. My observation at an academic institution is that more than 30 percent of the students are overweight. A study at a shopping mall indicated that about 40 percent of the adults are fat as are 25 percent of their offspring.

More than 75 million North Americans are overweight and are thus more susceptible to a wide range of incapacitating illnesses including heart disease, diabetes, and high blood pressure. Each pound overweight increases the probability of premature death by at least 1 percent. A person 25 pounds overweight has at least a 25 percent greater probability of an early death than a person who is not overweight. Each 2 pounds overweight ages a person 1 year. A person 20 pounds overweight looks 10 years older than his or her actual age.

Early death for millions of people is a result of the obesity problem. Obesity is also affecting the growth and development of nations. Excess weight is crippling the free world. Physical weakness, related to obesity, makes us an easier target for our enemies. Our capability to remain strong, to grow, and possibly even to survive may well depend on how we cope with the epidemic of obesity and obesity-stimulated diseases.

Fat fever is similar, in many respects, to the common cold. We do not appear to have a real cure for either one, so we spend billions of dollars treating the symptoms.

• Cold sufferers gobble up a wide assortment of pills, syrups, and other remedies until the symptoms are relieved.

• Fat fever sufferers try one diet after another in addition to using a wide variety of diet aids. Some diets reduce the overweight symptom but do not cure the illness. Unfortunately, 95 percent of the dieters gain back the lost weight shortly after the diet is ended.

For 20 years, I was 25 to 30 pounds overweight and suffered through dozens of diets and diet aids.

• I ate spinach and eggs twice daily until the mention of the words turned my stomach.

• I tried high protein and steak diets until steak became a punishment rather than a treat.

• I counted calories until I hated rabbit food.

• I used almost every advertised diet aid until I could no longer stomach the candies, cookies, and chalky dairy-type drinks.

• I drank corn oil before each meal for a month. It did little for my weight but created anal havoc.

• I even tried the drinking man's diet, which I must admit was somewhat more enjoyable.

I lost some weight while I was on the diets but regressed to my fat old self once I dropped the diets. It seemed that I was destined to continual dieting or everlasting corpulence. Fortunately, I became interested in the transactional analysis model for understanding human behavior and for analyzing our various selves, the communications between people, our life positions, and our life programs. Transactional analysis emphasizes that we have control of ourselves, we can think for ourselves and make our own decisions, and that we can change ourselves if we desire to do so.[1] As I read, studied, and listened, I came to the conclusion that from early childhood people are programmed to be fat. I reasoned that through investigation of a person's family and life pattern, fat fever causes could be identified which would in turn lead to discovery of the psychological and behavioral adjustments necessary to support a continuing cure for fat fever.

Eric Berne[2] postulated that a "winner" or "loser" life plan or "script" depends on early childhood decisions which are influenced by parental provocations and prescriptions. A fat fever program is a loser script. Hogie Wyckoff[3] describes the fat woman's banal script as a lifetime hassle between diets and scales. Overweight people who learn to like their bodies as they are and are assertive about their rights may reduce their loser feelings but do not reach winner status. They settle into the middle ground, a nonloser position. It is more desirable and more practical to maintain an appropriate, healthy, winner condition.

The story of Pandora's box describes the plight of most fat fever sufferers. The gods created Pandora, the first woman, to retaliate against man for accepting the stolen divine fire from the chariot of the sun. The gods reasoned that woman would plague, harry, and torment man. Pandora was dispatched to earth with a gold box which contained all the evils—hostility, disease, fever, hatred, intolerance, famine, envy, prejudice, gluttony, obesity, and so on—which have tormented mankind through the ages. In a last-moment display of compassion, the gods included one beautiful gift—hope. Pandora was cautioned not to open the box, which was a gift for the man who took her in marriage. Curiosity overcame Pandora so that she opened the box and the evils escaped to plague the world. Only hope did not escape before Pandora secured the lid tightly again. Most people suffering from the evil of fat fever relate to this myth. They resign themselves to the evil of everlasting corpulence because hope is still locked up in Pandora's box. We can open Pandora's box fully and allow hope to flourish. Eliminating the evils of fat fever through transactional analysis is possible for any person who has the fortitude to take charge of a self-cure.

The usual reaction to obesity is to treat the symptom by reducing food intake for a period of time. This solution is too simple for anything so complex as fat fever. The questions a person must answer are:

· Why do I overeat?
· How did I learn fatness?

The insights and exercises in this book are designed to surface the psychological and emotional issues responsible for fat fever. A permanent cure is possible only when you apply your brain to adjusting and eliminating your fat fever program.

Transactional analysis is an easily understood, simple process which uses common words in a special way. For ease of identification, the transactional analysis terms and some other terms with special meanings are capitalized. Thus when you see a word beginning with a capital (Parent), it refers to the special meaning. When the word is not capitalized (parent), it refers to its common everyday meaning.[4]

2
Cure Planning

RESPONSIBILITY

A cure is possible only if you accept that you are totally responsible for your feelings and actions. Others cannot make you feel good or bad nor can they make you behave in any particular way. You and you alone make the final decision! This is a difficult concept to accept because we are brainwashed into blaming others for our weaknesses. The young man who does poorly in college cannot blame his father. The young lady who gains weight cannot blame her friend who supplies the chocolates. The final decision to cut classes or to neglect studies was made by the young man in the same way that the final decision to have another chocolate was made by the young lady. We are influenced by others but the final decision is ours and ours alone.

Many obese people avoid accepting responsibility for their condition by transferring or projecting the responsibility to other people.

- I'm overweight because Jean cooks rich food.
- I eat dessert to please Sally.
- I wouldn't eat chocolates if Jack didn't buy them for me.
- I eat seconds because Paul hates to waste food.
- I have a couple of drinks before dinner because Tom doesn't enjoy drinking alone.
- If you weren't such a good cook, I'd lose weight.

People who take full responsibility for their feelings and behavior are able to say "no" to excess food without feeling guilty or sorry. This does not mean that a person will not have bad feelings; it means only that he makes the final decision about what, when, and how long to feel bad. People may duck their responsibility for weight control by projecting the responsibility onto someone else, but in reality, these weak people are saying: "You control me like a puppet; you pull the strings and I'll gobble up the excess food. As the pounds accumulate I won't feel so bad because I have someone to blame."

Refusing to accept full responsibility is a learned part of an overweight person's program. We learn to feel and act in ways which allow us to make decisions about eating and obesity and to blame others for our weakness. "Copping out" in this way is the action of a loser. I don't have to exert any effort to control my weight—I can eat, get fat, remain fat, and assume none of the responsibility. This is a good deal if a person wants to stay fat and has a patsy who is willing to accept the blame.

Often a wife, husband, father, mother, son, daughter, friend, or influential other person will try to assume responsibility for a person's condition. Forcing a diet on another person, policing intake, controlling and restricting food and drink, or cajoling, roaring, or insulting seldom works. The person may lose a few pounds, but the controller cannot watch forever so that sooner or later the lost weight, plus a few extra pounds, is gained back. When a person assumes responsibility for another person's obesity, there is little chance of a continuing weight loss. The psychological and emotional field in which the people operate is so turbulent during the periods of forced restraint that everyone loses something except weight. The principle of personal responsibility is the main reason that, under normal conditions, forced weight loss is not successful. A person who assumes responsibility for another person's weight control is wasting time and energy on an impossible task.

You are fat because you choose to be fat. You alone are responsible for your excess weight. The easy out is to blame someone else, but this is a loser's strategy. You will never lose weight permanently unless you accept the concept of self-responsibility and self-control.

The *Understanding My Responsibility* exercise is designed to get your "blame" feelings out on the table. I recommend highly that, wherever possible, you discuss, openly, your results with the person(s) whom you have been blaming for your weaknesses. It is important that you maintain your composure during this discussion and that you help the "blamee" to understand that a discussion of these issues is an important element in your cure. Once you identify and discuss the factors, you will realize that you are responsible; then you can move to change the pattern of your feelings and actions.

EXERCISE: UNDERSTANDING MY RESPONSIBILITY

1. Describe two events when some other person influenced you to eat or drink extra.

Event	Other's Name/Relationship	Why did you comply?
A.		
B.		

2. Describe two times when you ate or drank to compensate for an emotional reaction involving some other person.

Event	Other's Name/Relationship	Who made the decision to eat or drink? Why?
A.		
B.		

3. Is there a pattern to the events? For example: do they happen at similar times or under similar conditions; are the same people involved; are similar foods and beverages involved?

4. Place two chairs facing each other. Sit in one chair and support the contention that some other person or persons are responsible for your reactions to the events in questions 1 and 2. Next, sit in the second chair and refute the arguments that someone else is responsible and support the idea that you and you alone are responsible for your feelings and actions. This is a debate with yourself to air both sides of the issue.

5. Draft a short statement indicating that you accept full responsibility for your behavior and feelings.

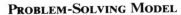

PROBLEM-SOLVING MODEL

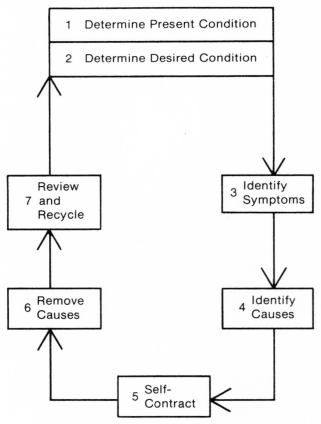

PROBLEM ANALYSIS

If food intake alone were the only cause for obesity, curing fat fever would be simple. Unfortunately, the emotional and psychological program is much too complex for a simple, intuitive solution. Finding an effective cure for fat fever is possible only if a systematic problem analysis is conducted. The problem-solving steps which follow are an outline of how to deal with the problem. This approach stems from the realization that a solution based on feelings and intuition alone is almost never effective and a solution based on fact alone is seldom effective. A continuing solution to fat fever requires a balanced integration of fact and feelings.

Step 1: Determine Present Condition

Determining your present condition is an important first step in problem solving. Specific quantitative and descriptive data tell you where you are now and provide a starting point from which to measure the changing condition. By using the following simple formula, determine an appropriate weight for your sex, height, and body structure. Please note that this formula does not adjust weight for age. It is my contention that it is a "cop out" to blame extra pounds on age. Healthy people with nutritional eating habits should be approximately the same healthy weight at 55 as they were at 35. The amount by which your actual weight exceeds the appropriate weight for your sex, height, and body structure determines your fat-fever-condition category of Warning Mild, Serious, Critical.

1. Using a piece of string, measure your least developed wrist directly above the wrist bone. A left-handed person measures the right wrist and a right-handed person measures the left wrist.

2. Determine your height.

3. Determine your appropriate weight from the men's and women's tables.

APPROPRIATE WEIGHT FOR WOMEN

Wrist Measures	Body Structure	Appropriate Weight		Adjustment	Enter Your Appropriate Weight
		Basic Weight	Add for Each Inch above 5' in Height:		
Less than 5¼"	Small	100 lbs.	4 lbs.	−5 lbs.	
5¼" to 6"	Medium	100 lbs.	5 lbs.	None	
More than 6"	Large	100 lbs.	5 lbs.	+5 lbs.	

APPROPRIATE WEIGHT FOR MEN

Wrist Measure	Body Structure	Appropriate Weight		Adjustment	Enter Your Appropriate Weight
		Basic Weight	Add for Each Inch above 5' in Height:		
Less than 6"	Small	120 lbs.	4 lbs.	−5 lbs.	
6" to 7"	Medium	120 lbs.	5 lbs.	None	
More than 7"	Large	120 lbs.	5 lbs.	+5 lbs.	

Example

My height is 5' 8". My wrist measures 6¼", which establishes my body structure as medium. Using the table for men, my appropriate weight is: 120 (8" × 5 lbs.) = 160 lbs.

WARNING CATEGORY. People within 4 to 6 pounds of their appropriate weight do not have a serious weight problem. This is a Warning. The extra pounds may be the early stages of a future attack of fat fever. A person at the Warning level has a fifty-fifty chance for a continued weight gain, a 5 percent greater probability of illness or premature death, and looks about 3 years older than his or her actual age.

MILD CATEGORY. People 7 to 12 pounds over their appropriate weight are well on the road to obesity and are suffering from Mild cases of fat fever. A person at the Mild level has an eighty-twenty chance for a continued weight gain, a 10 to 12 percent greater probability of illness or premature death, and looks about 6 years older than his or her actual age.

SERIOUS CATEGORY. People 13 to 25 pounds over their appropriate weight are obese and are suffering from Serious cases of fat fever. A person at the Serious level has a ninety-five–five chance for a continued weight gain, a 20 to 25 percent greater probability of illness or premature death, and looks about 10 years older than his or her actual age.

CRITICAL CATEGORY. People more than 25 pounds over their appropriate weight are suffering from Critical cases of fat fever. A person at the Critical level has a ninety-nine–one chance for a continued weight gain, a 40 to 50 percent greater probability of illness or premature death, and looks about 15 years older than his or her actual age.

Underline your condition category on the Present Condition chart and reflect for a few comments on the fat fever caution suggested by the category, the chance of continued weight gain, the probability of illness or premature death and aging. If you don't like what you see, resolve now to effect a continuing cure.

PRESENT CONDITION CHART

Condition Category	Pounds over Norm	Chance of Continued Weight Gain	Probability of illness or Premature Death	Aging in Years
Warning	4–6	50/50	5%	3
Mild	6–12	80/20	10-12%	6
Serious	13–25	95/5	20-25%	10
Critical	26 +	99/1	40-50%	15

EXERCISE: WEIGHT OBJECTIVE

Elements	Present Condition	Milestone Objectives					
		3 Months	6 Months	9 Months	12 Months	15 Months	18 Months
Weight (lbs.)							
Condition Category							
Body Measures Waist Hips Chest Buttocks Other							

Step 2: Determining Desired Condition

The desired condition is the optimum weight for your sex, height, and body structure established on the Weight table. It is important that you plan your weight loss with advice from your physician. Weight loss is a quantity success indicator. The quality of your success is measured by the ability to maintain your weight loss without on-and-off-again dieting.

The condition category of Warning, Mild, Serious, and Critical are useful milestone objectives. A 10- to 12-pound loss over each 3-month period until optimum weight is reached appears to be appropriate for most people. Do not set your objectives too high. An objective must be challenging and attainable. Now complete the *Weight Objectives* exercise.

It is helpful to remain aware of your condition during the weight control period. Symbolic items carried in a pocket or purse are helpful and the feeling, as each item is discarded as the milestone is reached, is similar to burning the mortgage. With instant cameras it is easy to take before-and-after photographs as you progress. Displaying the photographs in a conspicuous place in your bedroom, such as on your dresser mirror, is a useful aid to awareness and provides a feeling of success as you gaze fondly at the emerging new you.

Step 3: Identifying Symptoms

Weight and body measurements are the most obvious symptoms of fat fever. Other less obvious symptoms are speed eating; eating several times daily; eating before-bed snacks; consuming refined sugar, ultra-refined flour products, and other high-calorie foods in quantity; possessing a sweet tooth; eating to pass time; eating when emotionally disturbed; and physical inactivity.

Symptoms tell that you have fat fever. Treating only the symptoms does not bring about a permanent cure. Nevertheless, it is beneficial to be aware of the symptoms. Now, complete the *Symptom Awareness* exercise.

EXERCISE:
SYMPTOM AWARENESS

Symptom	Circle the Condition Which Describes You				
Condition Category	Normal	Warning	Mild	Serious	Critical
Waist size	Very small	Small	Average	Large	Very large
Hip size	Very small	Small	Average	Large	Very large
Buttock size	Very small	Small	Average	Large	Very large
Eating speed	Slower than all	Slower than most	Average	More quickly than most	More quickly than all
Times eat daily (meals, snacks, and coffee breaks)	Less than 3 times	3 times	4 times	5 times	More than 5 times daily
Reason for eating more than 3 times daily	Pastime	Emotional release	Ritual	Compulsion	Don't know
Calorie intake daily	1000	1500	2000	2500	More than 2500
Participation in physical activity	Never	Seldom	Weekly	Twice weekly	Daily

Step 4: Identifying and Removing Causes

Excessive eating is the energizer for fat fever and can be treated by sensible eating habits. Unfortunately, diets are seldom effective because they do not deal with the reasons for overeating. Most fat people know that diets are not a lasting cure but do not realize that their compulsion to eat is buried in their subconscious. Fatness is programmed from birth. It is even possible that the programming commences while a person is still in the womb.

A lasting cure for fat fever is dependent on removing the inappropriate messages which are programmed in the subconscious. Identifying the program and becoming aware of the messages is a prelude to a solution. Awareness and thoughtful analysis tend to decrease the force of some messages while others may need more in-depth work. Deprogramming requires intensive and possibly disturbing recall of the past, but a permanent cure for fat fever is worth the effort. This step will be emphasized in the remainder of this book.

Step 5: Self-Contract

A contract is a commitment to yourself to change a feeling, a behavior, or a psychosomatic issue or illness. A cure for fat fever requires a contract which includes the following:
  • Agreement to learn the transactional analysis language
  • Analysis of present condition
  • Objectives and schedule of events
  • Examination of your life pattern through the exercises in this book
  • Decision on what to change
  • Review and recycle at intervals

The information generated through doing the exercises will be the basis for a self-contract which will be finalized in the last chapter.

Step 6: Review and Recycle

Fat fever is a serious illness which requires periodic self-reexamination, much like the checkup from a physician after an illness or operation.

Review this book's contents and your exercise responses every 3 months until you are satisfied that you have coped with the psychological and behavioral changes needed for your permanent cure.

3
Drives

RECOGNITION

Recognition is one of the most important human drives. We structure our activities to meet our desire for physical touching (pats, hugs, kisses, etc.) and nonphysical stimuli (smiles, gestures, words, etc.). "Stroke" is the transactional analysis term for these units of recognition. Strokes say, "I know you are there and I know you are important or unimportant." [1]

From early childhood, we learn the type of behavior which achieves recognition. The popular saying "different strokes for different folks" is a truism. In fact, we are continually setting the stage to attract the types of strokes which we learned to expect and which we want. These strokes may be warm, cold, or zigzag.

Warm Strokes

Warm strokes make us feel special. Warm strokes say:

- You're O.K.
- You're important.
- You're competent.
- You're capable.
- I like you.
- You're fun to be with

Warm strokes express affection, compliments, understanding, and interest, and range all the way from a casual smile to an in-depth intimate relationship. Warm strokes are a necessity for the development of an emotionally stable person.

Cold Strokes

Cold strokes make us feel inadequate. Cold strokes say:
- You're not O.K.
- You're stupid.
- You're incompetent.
- You don't matter.
- You're not important.

Cold strokes express disinterest, put-downs, humiliation, ridicule, and insignificance, and range all the way from ignoring to physical abuse. Cold strokes will keep individuals alive if they are deprived of warm strokes. A preponderance of cold strokes develops emotionally unstable people and contributes to physical illnesses.

Zigzag Strokes

A zigzag stroke is one that sounds O.K. on the surface but carries a hidden message. Zigzag strokes say:
- You're O.K. under special circumstances.
- I have conditions about how I feel about you.
- You are too stupid to recognize the hooker in my compliment.
- I'm not sincere.
- There's a sucker born every day.

Zigzag strokes appear warm but have hidden cold stroke conditions which reduce their value. Zigzag strokes include outright lies, false praise, distortions, flattery, and saying the opposite; they carry the subconscious message that the stroke provider considers that the stroke recipient is not completely O.K.

FAMILY PATTERNS

Each family has its own behavior pattern based on observable orientations.[2] Children observe, experience, and learn that their family's orientation determines the type of strokes which are distributed for complying or meeting the family's standards and norms. The child learns that pleasing the big people is one sure way to get strokes. The desire and need for recognition is translated subconsciously into a lifelong search for similar strokes; thus the family's orientation becomes a self-perpetuating behavioral pattern.

The family patterns are:
- Kitchen—food directed
- Bathroom—bowel directed
- Hurt—hostility directed
- Love—empathy directed

Kitchen

The Kitchen-oriented family is directed at food and kitchen activities. The small child gets early stroking for cleaning up all the food on the plate, which is normally more than the child wants or needs. As the child gets a little older, stroking comes from learning how to eat without assistance. The payoff is Mommy's zigzag stroke: "Daddy, come and see how the *good* boy has *eaten* up all his dinner by himself." The child relates goodness and eating, and the Kitchen pattern is tatooed on his subconscious as the way to get recognition.

Formula feeding is a Kitchen starter. Time and time again, a baby will push a bottle away to say "I've had enough," but the unsuspecting "modern" mother pushes the nipple back into the baby's mouth because there is still some formula left. The baby soon learns that finishing the bottle means more stroking.

The bottle-finishing mother speeds up the introduction of solid food and continues to shovel in more than the baby needs. These mothers brag about how early their children were eating solid foods as if eating were an accomplishment comparable to running a 4-minute mile. One young mother bragged that her 4-month-old daughter was finished with strained baby food and was eating the normal family meals. The child may not get into the record book for early eating, but this mother is setting the stage for record-book entry for girth or some other obesity-related accomplishment.

On the other hand, the breast-fed baby is allowed to push the teat away without a fight. The mother has no way of knowing how much has been drunk or how much milk is left. No one has yet devised a "do it yourself" way to see inside a breast to check the contents, although some zealot will probably try. Some mothers start out timing their child's breast feeding, but usually after the first few feedings the mother drops this procedure and accepts the child's wish to stop feeding. I expect breast feeding and formula feeding are equal in nourishment but the formula baby appears to be more susceptible to Kitchen programming.

Kitchen families use food as a physical or psychological punishment. How many times have you heard these old stand-bys?

- The starving children in Africa would love to have that stew.
- Go to your room; there'll be no dinner for you tonight.
- No vegetables means no dessert.
- You'll sit there at the table until every spoonful is eaten.

Using food as a punishment establishes a cold stroke relationship which creates a subconscious desire to eat. Some persons who cannot diet have not come to terms with their subconscious feeling about the relationships between food and punishment.

Fathers who earn their living by physical work unwittingly set the Kitchen pattern. The breadwinner gets his warm strokes for providing "three squares a day." He relates fatness to health and accepts the obese child as a reflection of his provider capability. He does not view his children as fat but describes them as sturdy or solid. The father works hard enough to burn off his calories while his children sit gaining weight in front of the television.

Immigrants and other persons who come from a "have-not" background tend to be Kitchen people. They follow the pattern of the laboring family but have one added dimension. They know what it is like to be hungry and will not accept wasting food for any reason. Their stimulation is, "I didn't have enough food so my children are going to eat up whether they like it or not." These "have-not" background people often turn to physical punishment to force a child to eat.

The physical punishments range from slaps to serious child battering. One immigrant father dragged his daughter Sally to the kitchen sink and poured the unfinished plate of food over her head and rubbed it into her hair while yelling, "I'll show you what kids get when they waste food in my house." Sally, now in her fifties, follows the pattern. She is an exceptional cook and plies her family and guests with deliciously prepared food. "Have more" is a continual chant at her table. She is seeking and getting strokes for her ability in the kitchen.

Only one parent in a family needs to be Kitchen oriented to do the damage. A Kitchen father provides warm strokes to his non-Kitchen wife for her cooking ability. The young pleaser wife soon learns that receiving warm strokes is related to the richness of her table; thus unwittingly she reinforces the Kitchen pattern. These non-Kitchen wives gain weight but seem to reduce at will while Daddy and the kids continue to pile on the blubber. The ability of non-Kitchen people to take off and keep off excess weight lies in their subconscious or psychological reaction to food.

Many Kitchen-oriented women trim off excess weight at about 16 to 20 years of age because of their mating instincts. After a few years of married life, they revert to their old eating pattern. They gain the lost weight back and then sit around and wonder where the "fireworks" went. The easy answer is to force the Kitchen pattern on the husband and children, as misery loves company. Some weak non-Kitchen husbands may go along with the food bombardment, but a great many others turn their gazes to slimmer pastures.

Children who are unlucky enough to have two Kitchen parents have three strikes against them before they get to bat. Their psychological and emotional makeup is programmed for a lifetime of fat fever. These children have inherited a program for a disease as deadly as diabetes or heart condition. The major difference is that they are also programmed to enjoy the development of the disease and can't find a cure.

Kitchen people are conscious about their physical condition

and are continually making excuses for their eating habits.

- I don't need this but it is so delicious.
- I had a light lunch so I can have seconds now.
- I'd better eat this as it will only go to waste.

Food going to waste is not a problem now with refrigeration, but people still use the excuse. They are right that the extra food will go to waist but not to waste.

There are some relatively rare Kitchen people who eat but do not gain weight. These people are physiological freaks. Paul is a Kitchen person married to a Kitchen person. He eats about 5500 calories a day, works in a sedentary job, and still weighs 135 pounds at 45. The rest of his Kitchen family is fighting a continuous battle with obesity. Paul rubs it in by comments about fat slobs and uses himself as an example of the opposite, not realizing that he is one of nature's freaks.

"Birds of a feather flock together" is an old saying which applies to Kitchen people. Fat people usually have fat friends. They hate themselves for being fat but find it easier to live with if they associate with other overweight persons. They compare themselves to the "beautiful people" and reduce the frequency of these emotionally disturbing contacts. Jenny was obese throughout elementary and high school and had had a series of obese friends. On going to work, she befriended a new set of overweight people. Eventually the mating instinct dominated her life and she lost 60 pounds. Jenny's boyfriends were all heavy. As soon as Jenny married, her old eating habits emerged from under her mating blanket and she regained the 60 pounds plus some extra. She finds solace in her obese friends who are all sailing along oblivious to the tragic outcomes resulting from obesity.

Kitchen people who have enough will power to beat their weight problem act like reformed drunks. They look down their noses with disgust at obese people and rationalize their attitude as stemming from concern for the fat people around them. Gestures and looks belie this noble pose, however, and the obese person is driven away to heavy friends who accept the status quo.

This retreat serves only to stimulate fat fever, as the patient really needs to be around people who are not obese.

Bathroom

Bathroom-oriented families spend considerable time worrying about and discussing bowel movements. The child gets an assortment of warm, cold, and zigzag strokes for the frequency, quantity, and quality of the stools. The child soon learns to "ooh" and "ah" along with mother.

Bathroom people have their own language, such as "do-do," "ca-ca," "jobbies," "potties," and other euphemistic baby talk. They brag about how early and how easy it was to train their children. Strokes are provided for bowel performance.

Some people who suffer from chronic constipation are essentially Bathroom-oriented but reverse their application by withholding bowel movements. Constipation is more often a psychological condition than a physiological condition. The young child reacts to parental pressure—to go whether he wants to or not—by refusing to comply. Sammy learns quickly that all those Bathroom people, hovering over him, show more interest when he doesn't perform; thus he learns to attract more stroking by withholding his "pottie" performance.

Some young children who are forced to conform to the demands of big people realize subconsciously that the only thing which they have any real control over is their bowels. They react to emotional and physical upset by withholding bowel movements. Persons with chronic constipation can often trace their condition to a continuing, serious, emotional upset during their childhood. People with chronic constipation may have experienced any of the following:

- Some form of Stroke deprivation.
- Feeling unloved by either Mommy or Daddy.
- Feeling unwanted—being referred to as "our mistake."
- Being an adopted child in a home with natural-born children.

· Living in an unsettled home with parents who fought and argued often.

· Growing up in a one-parent family as a result of the other parent's death.

· Witnessing an ugly divorce, separation, or abandonment.

· Being subjected to physical abuse or to other forms of hostility.

· Having an alcoholic parent or parents.

· Witnessing a serious, continuing illness of a parent or other family member.

· Undergoing a rape or some other form of child molesting.

· Experiencing continual embarrassment and put-down or other actions which decrease a child's feeling of self-worth.

Case

Bob felt cheated by Geraldine's intense desire to please and to be with her mother. Bob described Geraldine as a monument to the old saying, "A son's a son until he takes a wife,/and a daughter's a daughter all her life." Geraldine's father died when she was 5 years old. Her industrious mother worked 10 hours a day 6 days a week to maintain the family and spent all her free time doing housework. Little time was left for the required daughter-mother stroking relationship. Geraldine admitted that she had an intense drive to make up for the limited childhood contact and missing strokes.

Bob and Geraldine were surprised when I predicted correctly that Geraldine suffered from chronic constipation with periods of 7 days without a bowel movement not unusual. Geraldine admitted, although she had never made the connection before, that a truly warm stroke involvement with mother seemed to stimulate bowel movements without the usual laxative aids. I have met so many reverse Bathroom-oriented people who follow this pattern that I was almost 100 percent sure that Geraldine's childhood upsets and continuing search for the strokes of which she had been deprived indicated a lifetime of chronic constipation.

Most Bathroom people are fascinated by bowel movements. When Mommy and Daddy are no longer around to hand out the strokes, Bathroom persons stroke themselves or solicit strokes from an unsuspecting mate. Statements of pleasures—"Wow, was that ever a good job!"—or mate questions—"Are your bowels regular? When did you go last?"—are normal elements in the Bathroom person's conversation. Bathroom parents are obsessed with toilet training and rush their child to the pot almost as early as Kitchen parents are introducing solid foods. Bathroom people often leave a child strapped to a training pot or a toilet seat for long periods. They rationalize this action with zigzag strokes such as, "Mommy forgot you, but the good girl did a beautiful do-do."

Case

Some Bathroom people punish a child severely for an accidental wetting or bowel movement. Barbara has two young children and babysits for another two youngsters. When a child has an accident, she leaves the urine or excrement in the pants for progressively longer periods as a punishment. Although this does little to change the situation, it does create a number of skin irritations and infections. Barbara thinks that a young child will learn toilet training from this type of cold stroking. When all else fails, Barbara resorts to rubbing the dirty diaper or pants in the child's face, following the method she used to housebreak her dog. Barbara is so Bathroom-oriented that no amount of confrontation or counseling has changed her mind about possible repercussions from this degrading, inhumane, and unsanitary cold stroke. My early reaction was that this "rubbing their noses in it" tactic was not common, but lately I have heard about others who use similar punishments that are often a prelude to child battering.

The squeezers and pickers of this world are Bathroom-oriented. Bathroom people will spend hours picking and squeezing every blackhead and pimple on their body in a compulsive desire to rid themselves of impurities. Some people who are not primarily bowel-directed show some elements of a Bathroom pattern by squeezing and picking.

Hurt

Hurt families pattern their lives around hostility. Children learn the orientation from Mommy and Daddy, whose fight usually starts with cold strokes—"You fat slob!"—or zigzag strokes—"Of course I love you; I like all fat women." After the physical signs—yelling, cursing, throwing dishes, slapping—are dissipated, the combatants sulk until one decides to take the first step to make up. Making up is a zigzag-stroking "I'm sorry" act and often ends up with sex. Hurts rationalize their behavior with "Making up is so nice that the fighting is worth it."

Children learn that temper tantrums, anger, fighting, and other hostile behavior attract cold stroke reprisals which will be followed by what the child perceives as warm stroke forgiveness. Joey throws himself on the floor and kicks and screams, which initiates a spanking from Daddy. Later on Daddy hugs him and explains "I did it for your own good." This pattern is identical to that of parents fighting and making up with sex. Joey carries this Hurt pattern through his life and transfers it to his own offspring.

Hurts get a feeling of superiority from hostility and forgiving. A true Hurt enjoys physical violence and the feeling of power engendered by striking a mate or whipping a child. Most Hurts stop their violence short of serious physical harm to their opponent although the emotional damage is significant. The mate or the child gets a few scratches or bruises which constitute the price they must pay for the making-up strokes. "Making up is so nice" that the scratches and bruises are passed off as a fall or from playing with the cat or dog.

Unfortunately some Hurts lose complete control as rational beings and become sadistic (like to inflict pain) or masochistic (like to feel pain). They want to hurt and be hurt. These egocentrics are responsible for assaults, child battering, rape, causing physical incapacity, and taking lives. Penal institutions are filled with persons who are Hurt-programmed. Many potential criminal Hurts do not reach this level because they find other Hurts who are willing to participate. In one city, masochists can get their needs met by a telephone call to "Dial-a-Beating."

Hurts are attracted to other Hurts. When two Hurt-oriented people are in a group, they quickly get acquainted and seem to enjoy each other's company. Hurts entering a new group pair up as if they had a homing device. This may account for the number of Hurts who marry Hurts and raise little Hurts while they spend a lifetime beating the hell out of each other and making up.

Hurts usually display a plastic outer shell. Their hostile activities may be known to neighbors and close friends, but the masquerade outside the home is carried off to perfection. Hurts know that their actions could not stand up to public scrutiny and thus they camouflage their Hurt pattern.

Hurts are overly interested in reports of violence. They become walking encyclopedias on the facts surrounding each newly reported violent crime. Their descriptions of violence, to anyone who will listen, are interlaced with zigzag comments concerning how repelled they are by these acts while in reality Hurts are stimulated by both the reports and the discussion.

It is the Hurt pattern which draws crowds to horror shows and movies filled with violence. Hurts, no matter how suppressed and controlled, are consciously and subconsciously searching for some form of release. Stories and pictures of birds or rats devouring people or persons possessed by evil as well as displays of sadism or masochism are drugs to persons striving internally for ways to release their hostility. A few Hurts are stimulated to violent acts by such stimuli, but these reactors have such an overwhelming Hurt pattern that they would turn to violence sooner or later without stimulation. The majority of Hurts, with more control and possibly a less strong Hurt pattern, get the subconscious urge out of their systems by watching violence rather than participating.

Some unfortunate people unknowingly marry Hurts. A Hurt in the mating dance hides the instinct from the unsuspecting prospective mate. After they marry, the Hurt pattern surfaces.

Early arguments and fights, over some form of sadistic or masochistic sexual behavior, are common among newlyweds. A non-Hurt mate will rebel at these suggestions whereas a Hurt mate will go along with and even enjoy the new outlet. A non-Hurt mate can participate, refuse to participate knowing that the Hurt will go elsewhere for the outlet, or abandon ship.

Non-Hurts often feel that they can play "Beauty and the Beast" and change the Hurts' pattern, but this seldom works. Personal awareness and professional treatment may change the Hurt pattern, but few Hurts seek help; thus the beast stays a beast. The "hanger-on" who plays a patsy role is being destroyed. Often the patsy will "hang in there" until a serious personal beating or abuse of an offspring forces the retreat.

A non-Hurt married to a Hurt is similar to a non-alchoholic married to an alcoholic. If the patient will not get professional treatment, the mate has every right to kick the patient out of the house or to leave. No person is required to take the inhumane treatment handed out by alcoholics or by Hurts. Unfortunately, many mates wait too long and become emotional prisoners.

· I'd leave but what work am I trained for?
· I stay for the children's sake.
· Jack's sick, I owe it to him to stay.
· My religion stops me from leaving—love, honor, and obey means a lot to me.
· I'm too old to start over.
· Mom stayed with Dad so I can weather the storm.

Case

Suzy is a young wife who was revolted by Sam's violent nature. Sam was stimulated sexually by bondage and whipping. When she refused to participate, he beat her into submission. Sam laughed at her suggestion that he get professional help, saying that she was a prude who needed to be trained like a dog. Suzy locked herself in the baby's room whenever Sam showed the signs of a ravaging intent. When she did not come out Sam broke some furniture and eventually left the house in a rage.

One evening, he caught her before she could lock the door and beat and raped her. Suzy ended up in the hospital with internal injuries and Sam went to jail. Suzy had been a patsy too long. Suzy's reason for staying was that her mother had stayed with her alcoholic father and Suzy saw herself as a similar type of martyr. Her mother had failed to change the alcoholism of her father but she was sure that eventually Sam would seek professional help or that her pureness would change him. This is a "Beauty and the Beast" model which seldom has a happy ending in real life.

Love

Love-oriented families are empathy-directed. They are warm, nurturing, and caring. They recognize each member of their family as an individual who requires understanding and love. Loves use physical warm strokes to reinforce their nonphysical warm strokes. Loves show their affection openly by touching, kissing, and hugging.

Loves develop an inner sense about the feelings of others. They know when to be intimate, when to be helpful, and how to ensure that interdependence overcomes dependence. Loves steer clear of cold or zigzag strokes and recognize warm stroking as a mechanism for emotional growth and stability.

The Love family is easy to identify. The children spend a lot of time at home, which becomes the gathering place for their friends. Love parents trade privacy for people and see a home as a place in which to have fun. Love parents seldom complain about untidiness and go for the lived-in look. Although Loves would like a nice garden and lawn, they see a place for the children to play with their friends as more important.

Fred enjoyed his garden and his lawn was the envy of his neighbors. One day during a visit, I commented on the damage the boys' tent would do to his beautiful lawn. Fred said, "At first I worried about the grass, but on a tradeoff it is more important to me that the boys and their friends have a chance to grow and test independence by sleeping out. The other parents wouldn't let them put up their tent for fear of damaging their lawn. Georgina and I feel that people are more important than grass; anyway, seed and fertilizer will grow grass again. The tent is our symbolic people fertilizer which is needed now—children grow up so quickly that there is no second chance with them. We love the kids more than the grass."

Love families have a busy household. The rules are few and have been developed by and to suit the family members. Trust and understanding are the basis for dealing with each other. It is not unusual for Love homes to attract every child or teen-ager in the neighborhood. Cards and other games are a usual and at times ongoing activity as Loves do things together.

Love parents discipline their children when it is required but seldom revert to violent physical punishment or any act which embarrasses their children or decreases their feeling of worth. Love children become aware quickly, from friends, that their Love parents and home are special and seem to govern themselves accordingly; thus discipline is seldom a major issue.

Young children from a family with restricted Love patterns often attach themselves to a Love family. At first, these "searchers" are embarrassed or afraid to touch or be touched, but eventually they learn by observation and experience that it is O.K. to give and receive affection. The more the "searchers" enjoy the experience, the more likely they are to feel disloyal to their own family. It is not unusual for "searchers" to brag a lot about their family members while they are avoiding them or reducing the contact. Everyone has a subconscious need to be loved and to love, but only the fortunate love "searchers" connect with Loves and thereby increase their own Love pattern.

Love parents are supportive but must guard against the dependency trap. The desire to nurture and help one's children can lead to a dependent rather than an interdependent relationship. Children who get too much help, whether they want or need it or not, can be smothered by well-meaning parents. A mother's hovering over her daughter like a heliocopter does not develop independence and maturity. It is hard to let go, but Love people seem to know intuitively when it is time to back off.

Loves give warm strokes freely and accept graciously the strokes coming their way. Some people find it difficult to accept a stroke without making comments which reduce or "discount" its value. A warm stroke—"I like being with you"—discounted by "I bet you say that to all the girls" is not the approach of Loves. A Love would probably react enthusiastically with "Thanks, we do have a good time together."

Loves have sociocentric values. They like and want to be with other people. They know by giving and understanding that they can contribute to those around them. Loves know that being loved by another person comes from loving first.

Primary and Secondary Patterns

Every person has some elements of each family pattern. That is, each individual is partly Kitchen, partly Bathroom, partly Hurt, and partly Love. The major effect on our emotional and physical life is attributable to our primary (most predominant) and secondary (next most predominant) family pattern. The first reaction to pattern identification is to select Love as the primary pattern as Love is what we would most like to be. After reflecting on past and present behavior, many early Love selectors change to another primary pattern. This is difficult to do, but it is an important part of analyzing the present condition. Accepting the idea that the patterns are not bad or good but a part of you with which you can cope makes it easier to select the pattern which describes your behavior most clearly.

EXERCISE: PATTERN AWARENESS

The Pattern Awareness chart will help you decide on your primary and secondary family pattern. Reflect on your past and present behavior, then select the one statement which best describes your feelings about that specific family pattern. Circle one number only for each pattern to provide you with a quantified value for the pattern. Each statement has two numbers to allow you a high or low response to the statement which describes your pattern. Consider each pattern separately and in the order presented. You may find it beneficial to re-read the descriptions of Kitchen, Bathroom, Hurt, and Love family patterns prior to completing your rating.

Family Pattern	Does not describe me	Describes me slightly	Describes me somewhat	Describes me well	Describes me fully
Kitchen	1 2	3 4	5 6	7 8	9 10
Bathroom	1 2	3 4	5 6	7 8	9 10
Hurt	1 2	3 4	5 6	7 8	9 10
Love	1 2	3 4	5 6	7 8	9 10

Pattern Awareness Chart

The pattern with your highest rating (1 is low, 10 is high) is your primary pattern. The next highest rating is your secondary pattern.

Using the rating points from the Pattern Awareness chart as a guide, draw a pattern pizza to describe your overall orientation. The example is provided for assistance and guidance only. It is not good or bad. It describes a fictitious person with the following ratings: Kitchen 8, Love 5, Bathroom 3, Hurt 2.

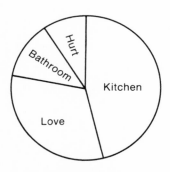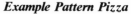

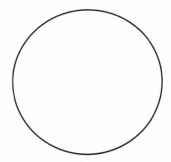

Example Pattern Pizza   ***Draw Your Pattern Pizza***

Every person has some amount of each pattern although it may be controlled or concealed. Primary Kitchen-patterned people are almost always overweight due to their subconscious relationship of strokes and food. A combination of almost equal amounts of Love and Kitchen can be disastrous. Mommy and Daddy see the provision of vast quantities of food as a symbol of caring, not realizing that they are setting up their children for a lifetime of misery. A combination of Hurt and Kitchen does not have the same effect on weight. The emotional trauma from a Hurt pattern often overpowers the Kitchen desires or possibly the resulting nervous strain and tension burn off the excess food. Many Bathroom-patterned people do not appear to suffer from fat fever even though they may eat considerately to provide ammunition for their most enjoyable addiction.

Generally, a person's major patterns will contain one of Love or Hurt and one of Kitchen or Bathroom. I seldom encounter a person with Love-Hurt or Kitchen-Bathroom predominant patterns, although I expect that this may be more commonly found by therapists providing clinical treatment.

It is not an easy task to change a pattern engrained in the subconscious. Once you become aware of your patterns, you are in a better position to make a valid decision on necessary behavioral changes. Curing fat fever requires a replacement of

Kitchen behavior. Some people making the change revert to bitchiness, sarcasm, and anger, which is increasing the Hurt pattern and is seldom useful. A successful and more pleasant change is to increase the Love pattern by providing more warm strokes. As you give warm strokes, you will feel better and the countervailing force means that you will receive more warm strokes. It is important to understand that the Love pattern does not include giving things another person does not want or need. Love is caring, which includes sensible approaches to food. Loving the people around you is a wonderful feeling, but it is also important to know that it is an O.K. feeling to love yourself.

The understanding and awareness you develop as you consider the remaining concepts in this book will provide more insights into your patterns. Feel free to revise your pattern pizza at any time as you analyze and gather more data about yourself.

4

You Are Six

Each person has three major personalities which are identified as Parent, Adult, and Child ego states.[1] The ego states are the sum total of a person's experiences, feelings, and learning. Everything that a person has experienced is registered in the brain for recall or reexperiencing. Sometimes our memory plays tricks on us and we distort the playback or perceive the experience as something which it was not. Although these distortions may mislead us, our attitudes and behavior are consciously or subconsciously linked to our recorded experiences. The source for your personal pattern pizza is in your memory-stored experiences and feelings which are transmitted in the present by your Parent, Adult, and Child ego states.

PARENT

The Parent ego state is characterized by the attitudes and behaviors which are modeled after the significant parental figures or big people who influence a young child. The significant parent figures may be fathers, mothers, grandparents, close relatives, close friends, or any other people in close contact with a young child.

I am continually amazed at the casual way young parents approach selecting a babysitter. People who study the consumer reports, test-drive several automobiles, and shop diligently before selecting an automobile choose babysitters with minimum investigation. They pick a sitter who seems O.K., whose price is right, and who poses the least problem with regard to transportation. They fail to view the sitter as a significant parental figure who may program the child to a greater extent than the natural parents. Some sitters are actually more competent at caring for young children than are the natural parents, and these sitters do a fine job, but others are less competent, even to the point of virtually destroying their young charges.

You are in your Parent when you talk, think, and act in ways which you learned from your significant parental figures. Similarly, your behavior and feelings are parental models for your own children and other youngsters with whom you are in contact. We say your Parent is programmed because you behave and feel like your parent figures without thinking. It is a form of learning which you use throughout your life. There are many fine things programmed in your Parent, but there are many other things which make you feel uncomfortable or are the basis for behavioral or emotional problems. You can cope with your Parent more effectively once you identify the elements of the two components: Controlling Parent and Helping Parent.

Young children adopt a whole range of eating habits from their parental figures. If Daddy eats quickly, Michael will eat quickly. If Mommy gets her strokes for cooking, Wendy will become a good cook to get strokes. If Mommy has a sweet tooth, Jackie will have a sweet tooth. If Daddy indicates that it's O.K. to be heavy, John will agree and gain weight. The saying "monkey see, monkey do" describes the copying child's desire to be like the big people. The Parent is developed as the young child adopts parental attitudes and behaviors which become part of the child's total being.

Controlling Parent

The Controlling Parent includes a set of erroneous opinions, norms, and standards which influence our reaction to life and living. Many of our opinions about sex, religion, politics, culture, racial issues, work, education, children, propriety, values, language, and, of course, eating are based on parental programming which may not be factual or complete. The generation gap, which many parents worry about, is often a young person's desire to question uncomfortable parental messages.

The Controlling Parent sets limits, forces advice or opinions on others, moralizes, controls, makes rules, punishes, judges, and criticizes. Example Controlling Parent messages are:

- Waste not, want not.
- Nice girls don't ride motorcycles.
- Men with shifty eyes can't be trusted.
- Women are too emotional for management jobs.
- Men are better chefs than women.
- Ladies wear skirts not pants.

The Controlling Parent structures a person's pattern of behavior, attitudes, and feelings about food. Forcing a child to eat, verbal and physical attacks over leaving food, using food as a punishment or as a reward, making a child feel bad about wasting food, speed eating, second helpings and consistent overeating, and stroking for eating up everything are some ways in which the Controlling Parent is programmed.

Much of the cold or zigzag strokes come from the Controlling Parent. The Controlling Parent is in gear when a person uses cold-stroke terms such as fat slob and porky, and opposites such as slim for fat. Controlling Parent zigzag strokes carry an ulterior message which say that the recipient is not really O.K. "I like to see a boy eat, but it's too bad everything you eat turns to hair" is a zigzag stroke from the Controlling Parent.

Our Controlling Parent forces us to finish everything on our plate, stimulates us to eat up the leftovers to avoid wasting food, directs us to eat dessert because it is a punishment not to have dessert, influences us to moralize about food waste, causes us to judge and criticize the eating habits of others, and in general sets the limits and rules about what, how, and when to eat.

We are our Controlling Parent when we force our children to eat "three squares" a day whether they want to or not and eat beans or spinach which they detest, send them to their room for leaving food, restrict dessert or mete out other food-related punishments, yell and scream about waste, force-feed infants, or punish physically for not eating. Rationalizing our actions by saying "I'm doing this for your own good—you'll thank me some day" is wrong. Our Controlling Parent is setting up our children for a lifetime of miserable fat fever, much as we were programmed ourselves.

The term "control" in the Controlling Parent ego state is designed to be a cold stroke. It is not coming from a Love pattern no matter how much we rationalize. The Controlling Parent approach to food stimulates a destructive Kitchen pattern. Real love is not critical; it accepts each person as an individual and takes into consideration that person's needs and desires. The body is a wonderful mechanism which signals the nourishment requirement to each adult or young child. We negate these signals from our Controlling Parent and fat fever is the outcome. The Controlling Parent can be reduced by replacing its messages with more sincere warm strokes.

The Controlling Parent messages control you personally and develop the Parent of those young people around you. You can react appropriately to the Controlling Parent messages about food only if you accept the fact that it is O.K. to say "no" to the Controlling Parent in your head.

Helping Parent

The Helping Parent is the part of us which sympathizes, nurtures, protects, provides, guides, and helps. We learn to be Helping Parents from the nurturing activities of our significant parent figures.

Everyone demonstrates some amount of nurturing behavior. Guiding a child about traffic safety, hygiene, and other protective limits is useful and necessary. Unfortunately, there are some people who have developed a smothering Helping Parent. These people do not know when and how to let go. Tying Jackie to Mommy's apron strings may be comforting to Mommy but can destroy Jackie's capability for independent thought and behavior. Most of us know at least one "Mommy's boy" who hasn't got it all together yet even though he may be in his forties.

The Helping Parent influences our food habits by making food freely available, overfilling the dinner plate, pushing seconds on the pretext that the food will only go to waste, providing food as a sympathy indicator when a person feels ill or emotionally down, and ensuring that a person gets more than enough to eat. We are programmed to apply these Helping Parent attitudes and behaviors about food to ourselves and to pass them on to the people around us. The Helping Parent says:

- Growing children need three full meals a day.
- Come on, another piece of cake won't hurt you.
- I always make extra pie for you.
- Cheer up, you'll feel better after you eat.
- Have more carrots and you'll be able to see in the dark.
- It's O.K. to be fat as long as you're happy.
- Extra spinach will make you strong like Popeye.
- Don't worry, she'll soon outgrow her baby fat.
- Every child needs cookies after school and a bedtime snack as well.

The Helping Parent is the most pleasant component of your Parent. It is right that you should guide your children and help people who want and need your assistance. It is equally important that you should come to terms with how your Helping Parent is influencing your Kitchen pattern. Your body knows what it requires as do the bodies of those people around you. Pushing food on others does not buy their affection; in fact, it is more likely to alienate them. People who push extra food, like those who coninually insist their companions "have another drink," are more often a nuisance than a blessing.

EXERCISE: MEETING YOUR PARENT

This *Meeting Your Parent* exercise is designed to help you identify the Controlling Parent and Helping Parent recordings which influence your Kitchen pattern. It may be difficult for you to describe your parental figures objectively. Most of us see our natural parents as perfect examples when in fact they had imperfections. Parents acted in ways which they thought were correct, for the child's well-being, based on their own parental recordings. You are not being disloyal when you identify the negative behaviors and attitudes of your parents. People are seldom trained to be parents. They learn from trial and error, and most parents recognize many of their mistakes. Who hasn't heard a parent say, "I wish I could raise my kids again, knowing what I know now."

Some unfortunate people have such a confused Parent ego state that they need to seek professional counseling to turn off their Parent recordings and to "reparent" themselves more appropriately. The need for total reparenting in relation to weight control is rare, although there are some people who need to devote the time involved in this kind of analysis.

Some people experience a blocked position when they are reviewing their significant parental figures. If you find that this happens to you, the block can be removed by reminding yourself that the information is for your use only and is necessary for an understanding of your patterns. A continuing change in your attitudes and behavior is dependent on complete background information, which includes an analysis of parental inputs.

Think back to your childhood and identify those big people (significant parental figures) with whom you were often in contact. You probably have a list of several names. Narrow the list down to the one male and the one female who were usually or often present at mealtimes.

Names of All Your Significant Parental Figures	Names of Your Male and Female Significant Parental Figures Present at Mealtimes

Some people have a one-sided Parent ego state; these are people who were raised in a one-parent family as a result of a parent's death, a divorce, or some other form of separation. Fathers who arrive home in the evenings after the children go to bed or travel extensively on business also contribute to a child's developing a one-sided Parent. The one-sided Parent develops when the absentee natural parent is not replaced by another big person such as the legendary "sleep-over Uncle Charlie." If you have a one-sided Parent, complete the exercise by considering only the one significant parental figure whom you have identified.

The following instructions will assist you in completing this exercise.

1. Complete columns 1, 2, and 3 of Part I (female parental figure) before completing columns 1, 2, and 3 of Part II (male parental figure).

2. In column 1, enter your answers to each question. Do not generalize. Provide specific answers with examples.

3. Consider each answer and determine how this attitude or behavior surfaces in your own Parent ego state. In column 2 identify this as Controlling Parent (CP) or Helping Parent (HP) input into your own Parent ego state.

4. In column 3 determine whether each answer is an input to developing Kitchen, Bathroom, Hurt, or Love patterns. You may have two patterns identified for some items—for example, physical violence over food may be an input to both Kitchen and Hurt patterns.

5. Leave column 4 blank. We will come back to complete column 4 when we are considering your Child ego state.

PART I: MEETING YOUR PARENT

Significant *female* parental figure's name _____

mom

(1) Your Answers to the Questions	(2) CP HP	(3) Pattern	(4) How does this make a Child? AC, FC, LP
1. What adjectives describe this person's eating habits? (quantity, type, speed, manners, way of eating)	*CP*	*Kitchen*	
2. What is the worst and the nicest thing this person ever said to you about food or weight? *food cook use to be prettier*	*CP*	*Kitchen*	
3. What is the worst and the nicest thing this person ever did to you with regard to food or weight? *fixed nice sunday dinners*	*HP*		
4. How did this person use food as a punishment and as a reward? *as gift to friends eating out*			
5. How did this person moralize about food, eating, and waste? *had to cut down bad diary day supply no much money no snacks pop*			

(1) Your Answers to the Questions	(2) CP HP	(3) Pattern	(4) How does this make a Child? AC, FC, LP
6. How did this person prescribe eating when you were sick or feeling down?			
7. What do you perceive as this person's primary and secondary pattern—Kitchen, Bathroom, Hurt, Love?			
8. How did this person describe overweight family members?			
9. Was this person a good cook? Did she provide more food than was needed? Did she provide high-calorie enriched foods and sweets?			

(1) Your Answers to the Questions	(2) CP HP	(3) Pattern	(4) How does this make a Child? AC, FC, LP
10. Did this person ever punish you physically or emotionally for not eating?			
11. What rules, guidelines, limits, and laws did this person set about food and eating?			
12. How were the rules and rituals enforced?			

PART II: MEETING YOUR PARENT

Significant *male* parental figure's name _____

(1) Your Answers to the Questions	(2) CP HP	(3) Pattern	(4) How does this make a Child? AC, FC, LP
1. What adjectives describe this person's eating habits? (quantity, type, speed, manners, way of eating)			

(1) Your Answers to the Questions	(2) CP HP	(3) Pattern	(4) How does this make a Child? AC, FC, LP
2. What is the worst and the nicest thing this person ever said to you about food or weight?			
3. What is the worst and the nicest thing this person ever did to you with regard to food or weight?			
4. How did this person use food as a punishment and as a reward?			
5. How did this person moralize about food, eating, and waste?			
6. Did this person prescribe eating when you were sick or feeling down?			

(1) Your Answers to the Questions	(2) CP HP	(3) Pattern	(4) How does this make a Child? AC, FC, LP
7. What was this person's primary and secondary pattern—Kitchen, Bathroom, Hurt, Love?			
8. How did this person describe overweight family members?			
9. Did this person get warm strokes from being a breadwinner?			
10. Did this person ever punish you physically or emotionally for not eating?			
11. What rules, guidelines, limits, and laws did this person set about food and eating?			
12. How were the rules and rituals enforced?			

EXERCISE: PARENT REVIEW

1. Review your pattern pizza in Chapter 3 and make any changes to your perceived pattern warranted by the recall stimulated by this exercise.

2. Make a list of seven negative fat-fever-related attitudes and/or behaviors attributed to your parental programming which serve your Parent ego state.

Negative Attitudes and Behavior	Corrective Action
1 eat vegetables before dessert	
2 eat quickly as example	
3 encourage fast food	
4 make huge quantities	
5 criticize manners	
6 only fix liked veg.	
7	

Outline a corrective action for changing each negative attitude and behavior. You may find it beneficial to consider how you can replace any strokes related to food with other warm strokes. Now, make a contract with yourself to adopt these corrective actions.

Caution

Remember, you are responsible for your feelings and actions. Your parental tapes set the stage, but you made the final choice to go along with the program. It is probable that you were uncomfortable but did not change because the cause was obscured in your subconscious. This book and its exercises are designed to surface the information so that you can deal with it objectively. Refrain from discussing your exercises' results with your natural parents; no matter how understanding they may be, parents can be hurt deeply by any suggestion of criticism of their parent role. Transactional analysis provides you with a model for self-analysis. It does not give you the right to hurt or blame others. Your parents cannot withdraw the program; only you can do the deprogramming and contract to make the changes. Do not blame your parents—you and you alone are responsible for your present condition.

CHILD

When you behave and feel as you did when you were a little boy or girl, you are in your Child ego state. All people have internal recordings of childhood experiences and feelings which are the program for their Child. The way a young child adapts to the parental messages is a further input to the program. One can say that the Parent "hooks" the Child.

The Child is conforming, fun-loving, angry, mean, spontaneous, affectionate, trusting, joyful, adventurous, creative, rebellious, curious, inquisitive, selfish, manipulative, whining, fearful, indulgent, and self-oriented. You can cope with your Child more effectively once you identify the elements of its three components: Adapted Child, Free Child, and Little Professor.

Adapted Child

The Adapted Child is the trained child. It is that part of all of us which reacts compliantly to authority, direction, and control.

A portion of this adaptation is rational and essential. One has only to be in contact with an overactive or hyperactive child to understand the value of some adaptation. Parental messages concerning manners, right and wrong, sociability, and safety, which are requirements in our society, are recorded in the Adapted Child.

Unfortunately few parental figures limit their programming to the rational; thus a portion of this adaptation is repressive to the development of personality. Example repressive messages are:

- You can get your own way through anger or hostility.
- To hell with the other guy.
- Pull up the rope, Jack, I'm on board.
- Little men don't cry.
- Children are seen but not heard.
- Shut up.
- Eat up.

The young child reacts like a robot, complying with irrational rules to avoid pain. The young child adapts to the behavior which gets the maximum payoff from the significant big people. If being quiet gets a payoff, the young child is quiet. If anger, screaming, and temper tantrums get a payoff, the young child is hostile. These repressive adaptations carry on through life and come out time and time again in our ego-state responses to similar situations.

A young child soon learns how to cope with messages about food. As Mommy and Daddy give strokes for eating, the Adapted Child strives to please by eating more and more. Many excessive eaters started out to please the big people and were hooked into a lifetime of compulsive eating.

The father who gets his strokes from being a breadwinner and reacts positively to his fat children is also developing the Adapted Child. His youngsters may feel and know that they don't want to eat more, but they comply with the message, often reinforced by Mommy, "When you eat up you please Daddy, who works so hard to provide you with the best of everything."

A young child soon realizes that big people can inflict punishment on little people if they are picky eaters, leave or waste food, feed unwanted food to the dog under the table, or reject certain foods, such as spinach, which the big people seldom eat but say is good for growing children. Pain and punishment are avoided by adapting to the repressive messages.

Recently, while driving to Montreal with a client, Dave, we stopped for lunch at a small restaurant. The only available vegetable was broccoli, which he declined. As the waitress put his plate down, Dave said, "I don't want broccoli." Her reply was, "Eat it, it's good for you." He dutifully complied by cleaning up all the food on his plate including the broccoli. As we continued our trip, I raised the broccoli issue:

- "Dave, did you enjoy the broccoli?"
- "I hate broccoli."
- "Why did you eat it?"
- "Damned if I know. She said to eat it and I did."
- "Did the waitress remind you of anyone?"
- "Aunt Martha, my mother's maiden aunt, rapped my knuckles when I refused vegetables."

Dave's reasoning said "no broccoli," but his Adapted Child said "comply or else."

Procrastinating over actions to reduce weight is an Adapted Child response. Fat fever sufferers who say "I must do something about my weight" or "I'll soon have to diet" are stalling. By putting things off, the Child is not defying the Parent and yet is meeting an internal, rebellious need. As a young child finds that stalling is successful, procrastination becomes a characteristic of the Adapted Child. The person who always says, "I'll start reducing next month," is a fat fever victim under control of the Adapted Child.

Some of the adaptations programmed in the Adapted Child are harmless; some are essential and helpful, but too many that deal with the Kitchen pattern are destructive and debilitating. Your Adapted Child may be destroying your chance for health, happiness, and the O.K. feeling which every person deserves.

Free Child

Children are born to be natural and free. You are in your Free Child when you feel and act like an unfettered baby which has not been programmed yet. Unfortunately, most people restrict the Free Child impulses which are the most enjoyable part of the personality.

The Free Child is curious, inquisitive, adventurous, trusting, fun-loving, aggressive, joyful, spontaneous, impulsive, affectionate, warm, fearful, and self-oriented.

The Free Child has no age. Some children learn to be stoic and serious at five years of age while others learn to have and use an active, fun-loving Free Child until the day they die. My children still remember and even brag about their "fun Grandpa," who at 70 years of age showed them how to do cartwheels and stand on their heads.

Children are bombarded with many messages which smother the Free Child, such as "work hard," "be serious," "don't be childish," "grow up," "curiosity killed the cat," "don't cry," and "get on the ball." Often when our Free Child emerges, the Parent steps in and says, "Stop, don't be foolish, someone will laugh at you."

Many of us miss out on the beautiful, natural, Free Child experiences because of a program which says, "Don't please yourself—do things which are acceptable and pleasing to other people." The truth is that those fortunate people who know how to have fun, can laugh at themselves, are interested in life, and laugh and cry unashamedly, when it is appropriate, please others without adapting to the unwritten rules of behavior.

The newborn baby eats to meet its physiological needs. Left to making its own decisions, a baby would not eat on a schedule. The schedule is more for the mother and the producers of baby foods than it is for the baby. The scheduling continues as the child grows until we are eventually programmed to have three meals daily plus a number of coffee breaks and snacks. This adapted eating behavior is not necessary for most people and is especially damaging for people in sedentary occupations.

Those people with a very active and open Free Child seldom

have a weight problem. They can walk away from food without feeling guilty. In reality, these people are comfortable in saying "no" to their Parent.

Fat people do not have a true Free Child. In fact, the jolly fat man is the product of authors and entertainers. There are few, if any, fat people who enjoy corpulence as depicted in "The Dumplings" comic strip. It is amusing to read about the antics of an obese couple, but it is not funny to live the parts in real life.

Fat people pretend jolliness to meet society's perception of how fat people should behave. They adapt to meet the rule that if one decides to be fat, one must also appear jolly. Fat people may masquerade their Adapted Child, but their inner feelings are not those of a fun-loving Free Child. Fat people are miserable, unhappy, and often psychotic about their condition. Fat people who pretend joyfulness and happiness are a pathetic sight. Hiding behind a mask of blubber may be some solace, but they are fooling only themselves. There are 70 million North Americans who know, by experience, that fat fever is not something to be happy about.

Obese people spend a lot of time fantasizing about what it would be like to be one of the beautiful people. The overweight female who daydreams about Prince Charming sweeping her up and carrying her willowy body off to a secret rendezvous or the obese male who dreams about his Mr. America physique on the beach surrounded by beautiful, bikini-clad women are fantasizing in their Free Child. The fantasies are some release from the frustrations and heartbreak associated with fat fever but cannot replace reality. When the dream is over fat people are still fat. Fat fever sufferers must accept that the fantasies in the Free Child and procrastination in the Adapted Child are working together to block a cure.

The way to deal with your Adapted Child is to say "no" and indulge your Free Child. Replace food, eating, and other related adaptations with fun and living for yourself and those around you.

Little Professor

The Little Professor is that part of the Child ego state which intuitively knows what to do to get the best response from the big people. The Little Professor is tuned in to the verbal and nonverbal meanings of messages, which allows the person to manipulate a situation to his or her best interests. The Little Professor is intuitive, creative, and manipulative. If you have ever seen a young person set the stage for Mommy and Daddy to fight, you have witnessed the Little Professor in action.

The popular comic strip "Dennis the Menace" describes the Little Professor. Mothers who bore others with long accounts of the wise sayings and actions of their children are describing the Little Professor. Every parent has examples of the Little Professor in their own offspring. One of the favorite pastimes for mothers and fathers is "My Little Professor is wiser than your Little Professor."

The Little Professor continues to operate throughout a person's life. When we are solving problems with hunches or intuition rather than facts, we are in our Little Professor. When we react to nonverbal signs, innovate, create, or manipulate, we are in our Little Professor. My 76-year-old mother is in her Little Professor when she switches her hearing aid on and off to control a conversation. I am in my Little Professor when I say outrageous things to test whether her hearing aid is on or off.

Kitchen people have a highly developed and very active Little Professor. It is the Little Professor which manipulates for additional food, sneaks food, pressures another person to break a diet, eats quickly to get the extra piece of pie, and uses the emotional response of others for Kitchen-oriented purposes. The following examples describe the Little Professor in action:

• Charlie and Sarah are dieting. As each TV food advertisement appears, Charlie draws Sarah's attention by comments such as "Wow—would that ever go good now," or "I'm so hungry, I'll never sleep tonight." Finally, Sarah breaks down and the pizza is in the oven. Charlie gets the food he wants and Sarah gets the responsibility for breaking the diet.

· Rob teases Louise about the size of the piece of strawberry shortcake she served herself until she leaves the table in tears or anger. Rob eats his cake, then finishes Louise's cake because everyone knows that the whipped cream will spoil if it is left too long.

· Molly's parents controlled the amount of sweets used in their home. Molly used her wiles to manipulate Mommy and Daddy into providing ice cream or candy by pretending illness or a down feeling. Molly continued her cunning ways after marriage so that Sam would feed her sweet tooth. Now that Molly is an obese 45-year-old, she blames Sam.

Persons who refuse to take the responsibility for their own actions and feelings and blame others for their condition are in the Adapted Child, but the intuitive, cunning manipulations used to hook another person's Parent originate in the Little Professor. Breaking manipulative and crooked patterns requires determination. Fat fever sufferers must become aware of their Little Professor setups and take firm internal action to stop. Say "no" to your Little Professor. There are many other more enjoyable and less hazardous ways to use the intuitive and creative parts of your Little Professor. Combining your Little Professor with factual data about fat fever will initiate innovative and creative solutions for cure.

EXERCISE: MEETING YOUR CHILD

1. Return to Part I and Part II of the *Meeting Your Parent* Exercise. Read your responses to each question and ask yourself, "How does this make a child?" Does it make an Adapted Child, a Free Child, or a Little Professor? Enter your response, (AC), (FC), or (LP), in column 4 with your reasons. This exercise will indicate attitudes and behaviors which need changing. As you are deciding what and how to change, remember that the Parent makes or hooks the Child. To change the Child you may have to change the Parent first.

2. Describe three common examples of your Adapted Child which influence your eating habits and decide on corrective measures.

Examples	Corrective Measures
1.	
2.	
3.	

3. Describe three common examples of your Free Child which influence your eating habits and decide on corrective measures.

Examples	Corrective Measures
1	
2	
3	

4. Describe three common examples of your Little Professor which influence your eating habits and decide on corrective measures.

Examples	Corrective Measures
1	
2	
3	

5. Review your pattern pizza in Chapter 3 and make any changes to your perceived pattern warranted by the recall stimulated by this exercise.

ADULT

The Adult ego state is the nonfeeling part of us which gathers data, plans, organizes, sets objectives, identifies and considers alternative actions, analyzes situations, solves problems logically, makes rational decisions, and measures results.

Fat fever sufferers do not use their Adult effectively. They do not analyze the situation or consider all the alternatives. In fact, fat fever sufferers seldom identify the real problem and thus spend their time treating the symptoms rather than the cause. The narrow approach of one diet after another, often of the gimmick or fad type, is an activity trap which has no lasting effect. Falling off the diet wagon is so frustrating and disheartening that most fat fever sufferers give up.

The Adult response is to reason out an alternative which will be an ongoing cure. The Adapted Child response is to stop trying to escape and wait for destruction. There is little chance for a person loaded with blubber to live a full life. Fat kills slowly but surely.

People unsuccessful at climbing onto the diet wagon say:

- Diets do not work for me.
- I count calories but never lose weight.
- As soon as I stop dieting, I gain the weight back.
- I must have a glandular problem.
- I'm always on one diet or another.
- I've tried every known diet; none of them works for me.

It is important that you separate facts from "guesstimates," opinions, and dreams. It is difficult to be objective about your "gut feelings," but your alternatives will be almost useless if they are based on subjective data rather than on reality. When you deal with reality you feel more secure in your analysis and eventual corrective decisions so that the probability of a successful cure is increased.

Use your Adult to gather Kitchen data by recalling your life experiences, by analyzing the present condition, and by observing others such as sisters, brothers, father, mother, your mate, and your children who learned from you. You can also get input from older people who enjoy recalling and reciting tales of the good old days, but remember that their input is likely to be colored by events in the intervening years and should be used only if you can substantiate its authenticity from your own recall or test its accuracy by consulting others who were involved.

Data can be gathered also by your Adult's sifting the information in your Parent and Child ego states. Each person, with the exception of the mentally ill, has an Adult which can do this job. Some people have better recall or more developed analytical skills than others, but every person has the capability to arrive at his or her own decision on weight. The assumption that one is totally responsible also carries with it the assumption that each and every one of us can make a decision to change and can effect a continuing cure if one truly wants to do so.

The data-gathering analytical phase is all important. No matter how hard we try, it is unlikely that we will be able to get together all the pertinent information. Often some useful input is blocked out by the subconscious. But if we work carefully at the collection of data, much information will eventually surface. Using the exercises for a group discussion is a good way to draw out additional information. The major requirement is to gather as much data as possible to serve as the basis for making a rational decision. The quality of conclusions reached will depend on the completeness of the input. In-depth information is needed because surface information is much too incomplete to facilitate rational problem-solving.

A person's Adult ego state can be highly developed in most ways but still be weak as it pertains to fat fever. Many brilliant people are obese. One wonders how people who seem to have what it takes to be creative and productive can be so lacking when it comes to dealing with obesity. It is possible that fat fever sufferers have a porous boundary between their Adult and Child and between their Adult and Parent. The Parent and Child take over to such an extent when food and drink are involved that the normal Adult control is smothered.

Many mentally ill people suffer from fat fever. Their Adult is excluded as a result of their mental incapacity so that all their reactions about food come from their Child and Parent. Mentally retarded persons are often grossly overweight due to Adult exclusion.

As a general rule, people who operate from one predominant ego state are inflexible. Too many fat fever sufferers who appear normal (whatever that means) exclude their Adult when weight control is the issue. Emotional and physiological reaction to weight-related things is programmed in the Parent and Child; therefore it takes a more rigid Adult to deal with the disease when it is getting or is out of hand. That is, the Adult has to take control to collect and analyze the data and to apply logic to a cure. This means an internal fight between the Parent, the Child, and the Adult. The Adult must be inflexible or rigid on weight-related issues and not give in to the Parent or the Child.

I am not suggesting that a person operate mainly in the Adult to the exclusion of the Child or Parent. People who use the ego state which is appropriate for the particular incident and time are flexible and feel O.K. The level of each ego state depends on the individual's program. Any one level is neither good nor bad so long as the individual is comfortable and performing effectively. The main point is that fat fever sufferers have an ego state level which, in respect to food, excludes the Adult. The Parent and Child responses must be replaced by sound and logical Adult input.

During the time the new pattern is being established, it is necessary consciously to use the Adult. Once the Parent and Child are under control, Adult responses to weight control will become a normal ongoing reaction.

Fat fever sufferers often consider that they are operating in the Adult, but in reality they are working from a contaminated Adult. The Adult accepts some Parent beliefs or Child distortions as fact and treats the contaminated messages as reliable input.

The Adult can be contaminated by the Parent.

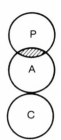

- Spinach makes you strong.

- Everyone needs "three squares" a day.

- When you are feeling down, eating makes you feel better.

- It is better to eat than to waste.

The Adult can be contaminated by the Child.

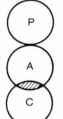

- I have to clean up all the food on my plate.

- Rejecting food is bad.

- Overeating pleases others.

- Eating quickly is O.K.

The Adult can be contaminated by both the Parent and the Child.

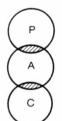

- Fat is O.K.

- Punishing over food is appropriate.

- Food should be eaten whether it is liked or not.

- Dessert and sweets are payoffs for eating.

The contaminated Adult, in the parental figures, is responsible for much of the programming which leads to obesity. It is easy to accept that the little people need direction, nurturing, force, and punishment in respect to food and eating habits. Rationalizing that children will suffer from some illness or incapacity if they do not eat a certain amount or type of food is an easy out. The little person adapts to the program and often never realizes that the less-than-factual parental messages are causing obesity.

It is the Adult which accepts that you and you alone are responsible for your feelings and actions. Even though you have been programmed in your Parent and Child, you made the decision to comply. Remember: you are fat because you decided to be fat. You can continue to be controlled by your Parent and Child or you can force your Adult to take control. This means a conscious decision to say "no" to your Parent and Child and to take full Adult responsibility. When you are stimulated by smell, availability, emotions, and the like, the stimulation is received in your Parent and/or Child. Consciously consulting your Adult and granting it the power of decision allows you to make an appropriate response in line with a cure. Your Adult will tell you that it is O.K. to listen to your Parent and/or Child in a particular instance but that it is also O.K. to reject the Parent and Child response. The Adult is the umpire between the ego states, calling the "balls" and the "strikes" by setting the ground rules for the encounter.

Each time you are forced by the Parent or tempted by the Child to consume food or drink, ask yourself these questions:

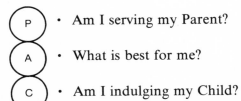

- Am I serving my Parent?

- What is best for me?

- Am I indulging my Child?

Case

Dick enjoys beef stroganoff and Jane has always prepared enough to provide him with a second serving. Dick attended a transactional analysis workshop and learned how to deal with the stimulation.

JANE: Honey, I'll get your second helping now. (Parent) *Dick's response depends on his ego state at the particular time.*

 DICK: Great, I sure enjoy your beef stroganoff. (Child)

 DICK: Good, we can't let it go to waste. (Parent)

 DICK: Thanks, I'd love to have a second, but I've had a good balanced meal and I'm at my limit for today. Let's freeze it for Saturday's lunch. (Adult)

Dick's Adult refereed between Child indulgence and Parent pressure by using the available facts. He also dealt with the waste issue and Jane's feelings by suggesting freezing the stroganoff for Saturday's lunch.

Dick reported to his transactional analysis study group that Jane's Parent continued to push second servings on him for a few weeks but that his Adult remained in control. Dick had been accustomed to having second servings on an average of four times a week, but he has not had a second for 7 months with a resulting 29-pound weight loss.

Jane changed her behavior of offering and cooking extra and Dick changed his consumption behavior so that he does not want or even think about a second serving. Their 11-year-old son followed Daddy's example and peeled off the 8 pounds which had been described as baby fat. Dick replaced sleeping in front of the television with family-oriented activities so that his Parent and Child are served in ways not related to food.

After 4 months, Jane joined the group. She attested that Dick had tried dozens of diets without much success and she hadn't really expected much from his new fad. But as the weight disappeared and he "burned the mortgage" by discarding his old self-concept and taking pride in the changes he could see in himself through pictures taped to the bedroom mirror, Jane became more interested. Although Dick was restricting his food intake, he did not seem to be dieting in the formal sense of the word. She wasn't preparing special food and he was eating everything. He was doing what he had described to her; he was revising his Kitchen program. Jane came to the group to learn more about the simple-sounding model which was changing their lives.

Jane has a Love/Kitchen pattern. She was nurturing Dick and her son by pushing food. She controlled her own weight by starving herself for a few days whenever she gained a few pounds. She was surprised to realize that she had not fasted for over 4 months although fasting had been a monthly occurrence. Dick's changing habits were rubbing off on Jane without her knowing it.

Jane is learning to reinforce her Love pattern at the expense of her Kitchen pattern. Rather than zigzag stroking with food from her Helping Parent, she has increased her warm strokes from her Free Child. This is not only enjoyable but is reinforcing Dick's changing pattern. After Jane joined the group, Dick's weight loss increased and Jane still has not fasted once. One may say that Dick and Jane have removed fat fever from their guts to their brain.

As we use our Adult, it develops the strength necessary to finish the job. We learn how to indulge our Child by some form of positive reinforcement and how to smooth over the discomfort in our Parent when we reject the parental messages. Transactional analysis is the executive model for this learning and individual or group education is the format.

Case

Carole was using fat-fever-inducing recipes acquired from her mother. Following the recipes produced delicious meals and attracted warm strokes, but all the family members were gaining weight. Carole put the recipes aside and used less fattening approaches to food preparation. She felt uncomfortable and disloyal but was able to smooth over the discomfort by preparing one of Mom's favorite dishes on each special occasion. Carole shared her mother's recipes freely with her friends and several were described in the local newspaper's women's page. This placated and pleased Carole's Parent ego state and her Adult was allowed to take control without an internal revolution.

Case

Peter found it very difficult to use his Adult constantly during the stability phase of the cure. No matter how hard he tried, he indulged his Child by excessive eating and drinking. Finally, we worked out a plan which allowed Peter to pay off his Child after set periods of Adult control. Each Friday for 2 months, Peter's Adult gave him permission to indulge his Child. Gradually, Peter lengthened the indulgence-free periods by a week at a time until he did not need to pay off his Child any longer. This transition allowed his Adult to take executive control and set the stage for an ongoing cure.

Most fat fever sufferers try to reduce their weight but usually give it up as a bad job. Typical rationalizations are:
- What's the use, I'll never lose weight.
- Even if I lose weight, I'll still be Plain Jane.
- I'm a food addict; nothing I do works.
- It's not my fault; Sally prepares the meals.
- I'd rather be happy-fat than skinny-sad.

Losing weight will not make a person a beauty queen or an Olympic athlete, but it can offer many people the opportunity to live a full, rewarding, worthwhile life. Any search for fame, fortune, or someone to love you must be approached by coming to grips with these truisms:
- There is no savior around the corner. You and you alone can take biological and emotional care of your existence.
- Learn to love yourself, then look for someone to love and you will be loved in return.

You are faced with the following alternatives:
- Eat yourself into an early grave.
- Hide in your room from the critical stares.
- Burst out all over.

- Stay drunk or high.
- Grin and bear it.
- Do nothing and wait for the end.

or

- Live in the real world.
- Energize your Adult and become aware.
- Learn more about and use transactional analysis.
- Gather and analyze the information necessary for the basis of a continuing cure.
- Decide on a cure program and contract with yourself to follow the program.

There is an old Nova Scotia story that goes like this: a man was walking along a country road when he saw a farmer working in a field with his dog sitting beside him howling. The traveler asked the farmer, "Why is your dog howling?" The farmer replied, "He's sitting on a thistle." "Why doesn't he get off?" asked the traveler. The farmer grunted, "I guess he'd rather howl." Too many fat fever sufferers would rather howl. You can get off the fat fever thistle if you really want to do so once you put your Adult in executive control.

EXERCISE: EGO STATES

1. Construct an ego state "snowperson" to represent your perception of the relative amounts of Parent, Adult, and Child you activate in relation to weight- and food-related issues. Reviewing your pattern pizza (Chapter 3) and the Parent and Child exercises (Chapter 4) will assist you. Section off the Parent and Child in a pizza pattern to indicate the relative amounts of the six persons in your head, as shown in the example.

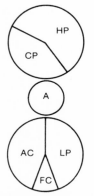

Example Snowperson   **Your Snowperson**

2. Are the boundaries between your Adult/Child and Adult/Parent porous when you think about food and weight? How can you put your finger in the dike?

3. Find a quiet spot with no interferences. Close your eyes and fantasize what it feels like to scale the diet wall.
· Does it hurt when you fall off?

· Stop and inspect the wall. Look it over from top to bottom, end to end and both sides. What do you see?

· Why have you never scaled the wall previously?

• Outline some Adult methods and actions for tearing down the wall.

4. You can decontaminate your Adult by considering the basis for your beliefs.
    A. List three words or phrases which you use to describe the factors related to food/weight.

Factor	1	2	3
Food is			
Diets are			
Fat children are			
Fat women are			
Fat men are			
Waste is			
Sweets are			
Hunger is			
Second helpings are			
Punishment is			
Eating rules are			
Eating habits are			
Cooking is			

    B. Cross off the words or phrases which you can verify/substantiate by fact. These items are Adult.
    C. Review the remaining words or phrases. Are they based on beliefs, old wives' tales, advertisements, experience, observation, or hearsay? Categorize as Parent or Child any words not supportable by facts to indicate contamination of the Adult.

D. Change each contamination to new words based on fact. If you get stuck try words completely opposite to the contaminated words. What did you learn about your contaminated Adult?

E. Which contaminations suggest fantasy, hope for a wonder cure, helplessness, frustration, anger, victim feelings, etc.

F. Answer the following questions:
- What did I find out about myself?

- What needs to change?

- What new Adult questions do I have to consider?

HARMONY BETWEEN EGO STATES

A permanent fat fever cure depends on the harmonious integration of facts and feelings. The transactional analysis decision-making process emphasizes:
- Decisions made on facts alone are often ineffective.
- Decisions made on feelings alone are usually ineffective.
- Decisions which integrate facts and feelings have a greater probability of success.

Feelings are the output of the Parent and Child whereas facts are the tools of the decision-making Adult. People who attempt to control weight by Adult actions, such as counting calories or restricting food intake, without considering the impact of feelings seldom reach a lasting solution. The result is a lifelong wrestling match between diets and scales.

Accord between the Parent- and Child-feeling ego states and the fact-collecting Adult is basic to a continuing, satisfying cure. Surfacing the compelling Parent and Child feelings which stimulate fat fever and applying the problem-solving Adult toward harmonious correction is necessary. It is not easy nor is it always pleasant to consider one's feelings analytically, but rational, logical Adult thought decreases the discomfort.

Many overweight people who are controlled by Parent and/ or Child feelings are on a rollercoaster toward destruction. Dieting may slow down the rollercoaster but it accelerates quickly as soon as the diet is discontinued. The fat-person hamartic, or tragic, life plans or scripts can be derailed by increasing the use of the rational, logical Adult. The person who digs deep inside the head for the source of the Parent and Child feelings and applies the fact-assessing Adult to determine alternative solutions and acceptable corrections can get off the rollercoaster. A cure for fat fever requires the conscious use of the Adult to plan reprogramming which will allow harmony between the Parent, Child, and Adult ego states.

5

Communicating the Program

TRANSACTIONS

Every verbal or nonverbal communication originates from a specific ego state and is directed at a specific ego state from which we expect the recipient's response.[1] For analytical purposes, it is too general to say that one person communicates with another person. It is more useful and specific to say that they communicate between ego states. In general terms, Bob transacts with Jean, but more specifically Bob's Parent transacts with Jean's Child.

Knowledge of transactions and the ability to identify and chart the three transaction classifications—(1) No Surprise, (2) Surprise, and (3) Hidden—is an important input for curing fat fever. In many cases, the origin of or response to a transaction is the executive order which moves fat fever on its destructive course.

Complete accuracy in analyzing transactions is not possible unless we have sufficient information about the sender's and receiver's ego states. Also, words by themselves seldom provide a clear picture of a transaction. It is necessary to include body language and sign language (tone of voice, gestures, expressions, posture, air of interest or disinterest, withdrawal, eye movements etc.) to understand transactions.

No Surprise Transactions

A No Surprise transaction occurs when the recipient accepts

a message in the ego state at which it was directed. The sender is not surprised by the expected response. When Sally directs a message at Sue's Parent and Sue responds from her Parent, as Sally expected, there is no surprise. The No Surprise transaction keeps communications open. Sue and Sally can continue their dialogue as if nothing has happened to block or disrupt the interaction.

A person can originate a transaction from any ego state (Parent, Adult, or Child) and direct it at any ego state (Parent, Adult, or Child) of the recipient. There are several possible combinations of No Surprise transactions such as Parent-Child, Parent-Adult, Child-Child, Parent-Parent, Adult-Adult, and Adult-Child. The measure of a No Surprise transaction is that the response was expected.

ILLUSTRATION 1

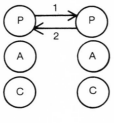

Mom   *Dad*

1. MOM (concerned Parent): Children need a hearty breakfast but Tommy refuses to eat his oatmeal.

2. DAD (stern Parent): He'll eat it from now on or answer to me.

NOTE: No Surprise transactions are illustrated by parallel communication lines.

Mom's Helping Parent stimulated Dad's Controlling Parent to threaten. Many young children are programmed into Kitchen patterns by Mommy's threat, "Wait till Daddy gets home."

ILLUSTRATION 2

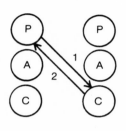

Dad   Tommy

1. DAD (power Parent):
Tommy, every boy needs oatmeal to grow strong. Now eat it up and no more refusing food, or else.

2. TOMMY (compliant Child):
O.K., Dad, can I use brown sugar?

Tommy's Adapted Child complied with Dad's Controlling Parent in order to avoid punishment. Transactions in which the Adapted Child is hooked by the Parent are a major input to developing Kitchen patterns. Seeking comfort or avoiding punishment through the Adapted Child becomes part of the ongoing program.

ILLUSTRATION 3

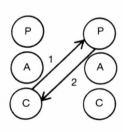

Tommy   Dad

1. TOMMY (whining Child):
Oatmeal is lousy stuff, it makes me throw up, and I'm not eating it anymore.

2. DAD (angry Parent):
You dare to disobey me. You'll eat it if I have to stuff it down your throat.

Tommy's Little Professor tried the throw-up maneuver which was met with Dad's Controlling Parent. Some parents do not pay sufficient attention to their children, who then become stroke-

deprived. Children soon reason that cold strokes are better than
no strokes; thus they may reject food to get attention. Using food
as a means to attract strokes is a Kitchen activity which is
common among fat fever sufferers.

ILLUSTRATION 4

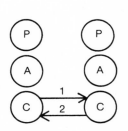

Dad   **Tommy**

1. DAD (manipulative Child):
The brown sugar soldiers on this side of
Milky River are the bad guys and the white
sugar soldiers on this side are the good
guys. If you can get the good guys to chase
the bad guys into your stomach in 10
minutes, your side wins.

2. TOMMY (joyful Child):
I'll drain the river first. You say "go."

Dad's Little Professor manipulated Tommy to react from the
Free Child. Eating games establish a pattern of consumption
based on the Child rather than on an Adult-determined need.
Winning by eating may make children happy and please
Mommy and Daddy, but in reality it is a loser input. The
contaminated internal message which says eaters are winners
stays with a person for life and contributes to the Kitchen
pattern.

Many grown-ups still play food games learned from their
parents. A few days ago, I observed my adult daughter and son
mark out their initials on a butterscotch pudding before eating it.
Wendy admitted that she did not really want the pudding but the
initial game, learned from me, compelled her always to accept
pudding. Everyone enjoyed the fact that I had also put my initial
on my pudding and was eating it even though I did not really
want dessert.

ILLUSTRATION 5

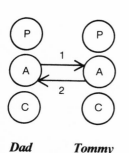

Dad   Tommy

1. DAD (information-seeking Adult):
What is it about oatmeal that you don't like?

2. TOMMY (information-giving Adult):
I like oatmeal O.K., Dad, but I get warm all over when I eat it just like poison ivy. Mrs. Smith said I have hives.

The Adult was used to gather data which would allow Dad, Mom, and Tommy to cope mutually with the oatmeal problem. Mom's farm family had oatmeal every morning and she thought Tommy was making excuses when he mentioned poison ivy. Later on, a visit to a specialist verified that Tommy was allergic to several foods, including oatmeal.

Tommy's mother and father are members of a TA study group. Nine-year-old Tommy was introduced to TA through Alvyn Freed's effective books *TA for Tots* and *TA for Kids.*[2] During one session, we were gathering information to compare Tommy's reaction to the oatmeal transaction with the reactions of his parents. Tommy said, "Some things hate you, but no one but you knows it. You can cry, yell, scream, and throw up, but you get a spanking and still have to eat the haters." Later in the session Tommy said, "Dr. Tully said to keep away from bees because bees hate me. If I don't like bees and bees hate me, how come I always have hives?"

How many people force their children to eat food which the children don't like or to which they are allergic? In a TA study group of 16 persons, 14 owned up to force feeding their offspring. Five people admitted that their children had become ill, yet not one person had considered the possibility of an allergy. Kitchen people do not seem to understand that individuals may react differently to specific foods or drinks. Pressing children to eat not only reinforces the Kitchen pattern but could constitute a serious health hazard in the form of allergic reactions.

Even very young children get signals about what they like or don't like and, to use Tommy's term, about what things hate them. All youngsters have a developing Adult from which they can explain their reactions to food and eating if we provide the time and have the patience to listen and probe for input. Unfortunately, the big people seldom listen carefully to children: the Parent tape says children should be seen and not heard. Kitchen people spend so much time listening to their own "eat up" music that they get out of tune with reality. Young children are people, not possessions, and deserve the right to be heard and to receive adequate explanations when their feelings and desires are out of line with the wishes of the big people. Persons with a combination of Kitchen and Hurt family patterns pay little attention to the rights of other people, and when the other person is smaller, Parent force and pressure replace the logical and rational Adult.

EXERCISE: NO SURPRISE TRANSACTIONS

1. Describe and illustrate one food- or weight-related No Surprise transaction recalled from your childhood. Comment on how this transaction influenced a Kitchen pattern.

Illustration   **Transaction**

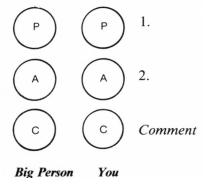

1.

2.

Comment

Big Person   *You*

2. The majority of No Surprise transactions, which are food-related, originate from the Parent and hook the Child. Think carefully about your transactions. Is the Parent in your brain hooking the Child in your stomach? The Parent hook is barbed like a fish hook in that it catches securely the hungry Child. Suggest two methods that you can use to straighten out the barb and escape the Parent hook in your head.

a.

b.

Surprise Transactions

A Surprise transaction occurs when a message does not reach the target ego state. The sender is surprised by the unexpected response. When Carl directs a message at Sue's Adult and she responds from the Child, the transaction is crossed and communications are disrupted. Communications close when the majority of transactions get unexpected responses.

Surprise transactions initiate emotional pain, violent reactions, yelling, fighting, and punishment. The Surprise transaction causes the Hurt pattern in people to surface. Behaviors, such as force, pressure, or punishment for food-related incidents, are rationalized as nurturing—doing something for someone else's good—but are really Kitchen/Hurt operating from the Controlling Parent. The Surprise transaction integrates force and food into one package in the program and transfers the pattern from generation to generation.

ILLUSTRATION 6

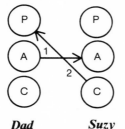

Dad   **Suzy**

1. DAD (information-giving Adult):
Steak contains proteins for developing strong bodies.

2. SUZY (hostile Child):
I hate steak and I won't eat it.

Dad's Adult directed factual information at Suzy's Adult but Suzy replied from her Child. Surprise or crossed transactions create a level of tension about food which prolongs the uproar. Dad can reduced the tension somewhat by originating another Adult information-seeking transaction such as, "Why do you hate steak, Suzy?" or he can apply force and pressure which is most often the case.

This could be another example of a stroke-deprived Child setting up a cold stroke encounter. Suzy could be saying: "I'm here; recognize me even if it is by a slap."

ILLUSTRATION 7

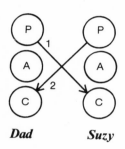

Dad **Suzy**

1. DAD (directing Parent): "Suzy, eat up your green beans, they're good for you.

2. SUZY (criticizing Parent): They are not—I don't want to be fat like you.

Dad directed his comment from the Controlling Parent at Suzy's Adapted Child. He was surprised by Suzy's Parent response. Surprise transactions tend to be personal and initiate Hurt reactions. Dad can initiate an Adult Transaction: "I have gained a few pounds lately. What do you think I should do about it?" This allows Suzy to deal with the food issues from her Adult, thereby reducing tension. Unfortunately, the usual response from Dad is yelling, threatening, force feeding, or even striking.

Fat fever sufferers are very sensitive about their weight. They may comment or make jokes about their condition but react violently to direct or implied criticism. A fat lady asked a shoe store clerk, "Do you shoe horses?" He answered, "We can shoe anything; sit right down here." A swipe of her handbag broke his nose.

The old saying of "count to ten before you act" or "turn the other cheek" are tried and true ways to defuse Surprise transactions. If we stop and think, we can consciously redirect

the transaction, positively. Continuing on by crossing the transaction is the start of a fight. Much of the assault and battery
unrelated to robbery started with Surprise transactions.

Many husband and wife quarrels are ignited by Surprise
transactions. Although some uproars originate from the couple's
own Hurt patterns, more fights start over the eating habits of
their children. When parents realize that children will eat what
they need without being forced, not only will the children be
programmed more appropriately but family life will be more
serene and pleasant. Mealtimes should be fun not misery.

ILLUSTRATION 8

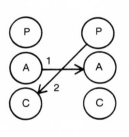

Mom   *Dad*

1. MOM (problem-solving Adult):
Pearl has rejected her dinner for three
nights in a row. What do you think I
should do?

2. DAD (critical Parent):
Can't you make even one little decision
without bugging me?

Mom was seeking advice but instead received a put-down,
and the fight was on.

ILLUSTRATION 9

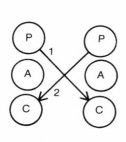

Mom   *Dad*

1. MOM (critical Parent):
You don't even care about your own daughter. All I ever hear from you is work, work, work. I'm fed up with assuming all the responsibility around here.

2. DAD (angry Parent):
Quit your complaining. Raising a family is all you have to do. I wish I had it that easy.

Fights which originate over the eating habits of children usually end up with punishment for the little person. Either Mom or Dad or both turn on Pearl with, "Every time you refuse to eat, Mommy and Daddy fight." Many Pearls of this world, of all ages, eat to please others and to maintain peace. When Pearl does not like, want, or need food, she has the right to be assertive and to say "no."

I remember times when I ate food to please my wife, Joy, but now we have an understanding that allows me to reject food without an uproar or sulking. Joy still feels a little hurt when I say "no" to food which she spent hours preparing, but she respects my right to be assertive about what, how, and when I eat. As Joy became attuned to the changing me, she adapted her cooking and food preparation habits to coincide with my new program so that now we are usually on the same track.

Reducing Surprise transactions about weight, food, or any other subject requires a new approach to dialogue where:

• Channels of communication are kept open by decreasing and defusing Surprise transactions.

• Conflict is not suppressed but mentally coped with in the Adult.

• Commitment is based on trust, not the power Parent.

• Feedback is sensitive and describes here-and-now reality from the Adult.

• Leveling is telling it how it really is while remaining cognizant of the difference between leveling from the Adult and flattening from the Parent.

EXERCISE: SURPRISE TRANSACTIONS

1. Describe and illustrate one food- or weight-related Surprise transaction in which you were involved.

Illustration

A.   1.

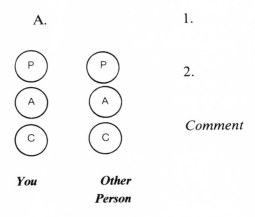

2.

Comment

You   *Other*
              Person

2. What responsibility did you have for this Surprise transaction and the results?

3. List three methods which you can use to reduce Kitchen-oriented Surprise transactions.

A.

B.

C.

Hidden Transactions

A Hidden transaction occurs when a crooked, ulterior message is sent. The transaction appears plausible and Adult but has a hidden objective of hooking another ego state. Hidden transactions with crooked messages are going on around us continuously. The door-to-door magazine salesman who says, "I was here earlier and your wife said these magazines were too deep for you," is attempting a Child hook. You may reply from the Adult, "She's right, I wouldn't read them," or from the hooked Child, "We'll take them."

Hidden transactions are a favorite tool of Kitchen people for disrupting diets, initiating fat fever activities, projecting blame on others, and generally raising hell about food, eating, and weight.

ILLUSTRATION 10

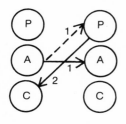

Joe   *Donna*

1. JOE (crooked Adult):
Do we still have that half-pizza in the freezer?
2. DONNA (nurturing Parent):
I can't stand to see you starving; let's have it now. One little break in your diet won't hurt.

NOTE: **Hidden transactions are illustrated by a dotted line which indicates the ulterior, psychological hook. This is not a crossed transaction because the real message is illustrated by the dotted communication line.**

Joe asked a question which appeared Adult but was designed to hook Donna's Helping Parent, expecting that he would get his piece of pizza.

Dieting Kitchen people have a sixth sense about how to hook the Parent or Child in others. When the other person complies by providing food, the Kitchen person has a patsy who absorbs the abuse for breaking the diet. People who look for and use a patsy have a major barrier to an ongoing cure: they have not accepted full responsibility for their actions and feelings.

ILLUSTRATION 11

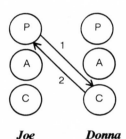

Joe   Donna

1. JOE (blaming Parent):
You knew I was on a diet yet you made pizza. My diet's all shot and it's your fault.

2. DONNA (guilty Child):
I'm sorry, dear, I thought I was pleasing you.

Joe blamed Donna for being the patsy and transferred his guilt to her. Donna, still playing the patsy, accepted "the monkey on her back" instead of leaving it with Joe where it belonged. Joe had the pizza which he wanted and was able to walk away leaving the guilt with his patsy.

Donna may have reacted from the critical Parent with a Surprise response directed at Joe's Child.

ILLUSTRATION 12

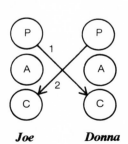

Joe   Donna

1. JOE (blaming Parent):
You knew I was on a diet yet you made pizza. My diet's shot and it's your fault.

2. DONNA (critical Parent):
Don't try to put the blame on me.

Donna's unexpected response raises the tension level and the fight is on. After the combatants calm down, Joe uses his emotional upset as another diet escape and raids the refrigerator. Most Kitchen people have a Parent message which says, "Eat when you're upset."

Illustrations 10 and 11 are typical of the way a Kitchen person hooks and blames a patsy. Illustration 12 indicates the progression to a fight when a person hooked by a Hidden transaction refuses to take the blame or be the patsy. Both approaches are Kitchen successes—in one he gets pizza and a patsy, in the other he gets pizza and a reason for further eating. Illustration 13 indicates a more appropriate response which leaves the responsibility with Joe.

ILLUSTRATION 13

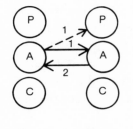

Joe   *Donna*

1. JOE (crooked Adult):
Do we still have that half-pizza in the freezer?

2. DONNA (responsibility-establishing Adult):
Yes. Remember, your diet is your responsibility. If you decide to eat pizza, it is up to you.

Case

Stan was an on-again, off-again dieter. As a policeman, he had to remain fit. On four occasions, Stan's superintendent had directed him to get within the force's allowable weight range or face disciplinary action. At a study group meeting, Stan described his attempts at dieting and Mae's actions which enticed him to go off his diet. Stan was provided some basic information about transactional analysis and family patterns. He was asked to consider carefully the concept that he alone is responsible for his feelings and behavior. Mae was invited to the next study session.

At the second session, the group disregarded Stan's issue and discussed instead how Claude Steiner's creative treatment for alcoholics [3] applied to fat fever sufferers. Eventually, Mae could hold back no longer and blurted out, "Stan's a food addict and I'm his patsy—no wonder I always feel so miserable when he's dieting."

Stan contracted to assume complete responsibility for solving his problem and to stop hooking and blaming Mae for his own weaknesses.

Mae contracted to give up the patsy role. This meant replacing some of her nurturing ways with Adult behavior. Mae agreed not to react negatively if Stan continued his Kitchen pattern. It was to be truly his responsibility. She would not shoulder the blame when he fell off the food wagon.

Mae and Stan remained in the study group in order to learn more about transactional analysis. Stan altered his Kitchen pattern sufficiently so that his weight stabilized at the lower limit of the force's allowable weight range. Stan admitted that this was the first time he had ever controlled his eating successfully. Stan knew he had won the battle when he was no longer affected by the eating habits of his younger patrol partner. Mae is pleased with the new physical Stan but is ecstatic about the effect on their existence which she describes as "a continuing honeymoon."

ILLUSTRATION 14

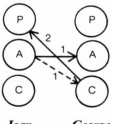

Joan   George

1. JOAN (crooked Adult):
Sally sent us a present of their spiced meat today.

2. GEORGE (hooked Child):
Wow, how about a Polish sausage.

Joan's Adult-appearing statement has a hidden hook to manipulate the situation so that their diet will be disrupted. After all, no one really expects her to sit by while George tastes the Polish sausage. George could have responded in the Adult, "That was nice of Sally—I'll call tomorrow to thank them," which would straighten out the hook. Instead, as Joan planned, his Kitchen pattern allowed him to be hooked in the Child.

Kitchen people are adept at casting out the line loaded with sinkers and three-pronged barbed hook. It takes an observant and aware person to straighten out the hook. When a fat fever sufferer accepts responsibility, Hidden transactions are less frequent. Responsibility means that Adult transactions are truly Adult. Input and feedback are direct, to the point, and honest No Surprise transactions based on the positive openness and leveling necessary for an ongoing cure.

Fat fever sufferers often participate in gestures or other inappropriate nonverbal signs which reinforce Kitchen patterns. Claude Steiner describes this destructive reinforcing behavior as a "gallows transaction." [4] The fat person who laughs about his condition is adding leg irons to the hangman's noose. The friend who laughs along with him is providing the handcuffs and restraining chains. Fat fever is not the least bit funny or pleasant. Destroying oneself is hardly a laughing matter. Nor is providing the zigzag "ha ha" strokes to a self-destructive person a pleasant enterprise.

ILLUSTRATION 15

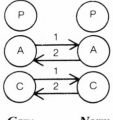

Gary   Norm

1. GARY (destroying Child):
I had a great time last night. Eleven beers and three plates of spaghetti. Ha ha ha ha.

2. NORM (reinforcing Child):
You did your thing. Ha ha ha ha.

The words are Adult but the ha ha comes from the Child. Kitchen people brag about the number of drinks and amount of food consumed as a measure of a good time. Gary's "ha ha ha ha" is tightening the noose and adding the leg irons while Norm's "ha ha ha ha" is the zigzag stroke which clamps on handcuffs and restraining chains. Laughing for enjoyment is joyful, but laughing to avoid tears is pathetic. Crying or showing emotion is neither a sign of weakness nor wrong. Fat fever sufferers may cry because of their condition but do not need to cry in desperation. The cure is around the corner for those who have the desire to make the transition.

Fat fever sufferers are touchy about gallows transactions, although they appear to get some solace from the manacle-providing laughs. In reality, they are hurt badly by the gallows-transaction reinforcement. Searching for truly funny things to enjoy and to laugh at is more friendly and beneficial than joining in laughter with the tragic fat person at himself and his Kitchen-oriented destructive behavior.

EXERCISE: HIDDEN TRANSACTIONS

1. Describe and illustrate one food- or weight-related Hidden transaction in which you were involved.

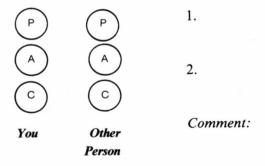

1.

2.

Comment:

2. List three methods which you will use to reduce Hidden transactions.

    A.

    B.

    C.

EXERCISE: TRANSACTION REVIEW

1. This exercise provides you with an opportunity to review how frequently you use or apply some fat fever factors in your transactions. Remember, your decision must be based on food-, weight-, and other Kitchen-related issues only. Check the appropriate column beside each factor.

Transaction Factors	1 Never	2 Seldom	3 Sometimes	4 Often	5 Very Often
A. No Surprise transactions					
B. Surprise transactions					
C. Hidden transactions					
D. Gallows transactions					
E. Uproars, generally					
F. Openness and leveling					
G. Adult morality-based feedback					
H. Parent power					
I. Gee-whiz Free Child					
J. Manipulation/hooks					
K. Cold or zigzag strokes					
L. Patsy					
M. Food games					

2. Choose four of the transaction factors which need improvement. Decide on improvement action. Pick factors which have an impact on your Kitchen pattern and which you can correct or improve.

A.

B.

C.

D.

6

Perpetuating Fat Fever

Fat fever sufferers play a number of roles based on a pre-programmed pattern. A cure requires identification of the roles and patterns so that corrective action can be taken.

FAT FEVER DRAMAS

Fat fever is a series of real-life "Drama Triangles" with participants playing out the three roles of Persecutor, Victim, and Rescuer. Although we assume a starting role in each Drama, the roles switch in ways similar to the unexpected action, response, or outcome in a good play. A life Drama has several transactions and role switches and one person may play all the roles at one time or another. It is also possible for one person to play more than one role at the same time.[1]

Case

When Kip arrived home at 6 P.M., 4-year-old Jimmy and his mother Sarah were crying.

SARAH (Victim): I wanted to get him fed and bathed before you got home so that we could have a nice quiet dinner for once. You work so hard. He just refused to eat and finally threw his whole dinner on the dog's back. When the dog spread the food all over my nice clean floor, I lost my temper.

KIP (Rescuer): I don't blame you for losing your temper. I'll mix you a tall, cool gin and while you enjoy it I'll feed Jimmy. We'll still have a nice dinner.

Sarah was setting up the Drama to rescue hard-working Kip by providing a nice quiet dinner. When Jimmy refused to eat, Sarah switched to the Persecutor role. Eventually the roles switched again and Sarah was the Victim and Jimmy the Persecutor. When Kip arrived home, he took over as the Rescuer, which was a complete switch from the opening intent.

A more usual Drama is "Wait till your daddy gets home" or "Woodshed."

SARAH (Victim): You'll have to do something about Jimmy. I just can't cope with his mealtime tantrums. I've given up.

KIP (Rescuer/Persecutor): Jimmy, go to your room. You have to be taught to obey, even if it means a spanking.

Victim Jimmy had felt persecuted by Sarah and held out on eating until Sarah's frustrated Child allowed her role switch to Victim with 4-year-old Jimmy assuming the Persecutor's role. Kip's power response was to rescue Sarah and persecute Jimmy at the same time, thus playing two roles. Jimmy was back in the Victim role, which is a normal switch for the little people. The Drama continued:

JIMMY (Victim): Don't spank me any more, Daddy, I'll be good.

SARAH (Rescuer): Stop this minute, Kip, you're hurting my little boy. I only wanted you to talk to him, not whip him.

KIP (Persecutor): Mind your business. Discipline is my responsibility.

SARAH (Rescuer/Persecutor): I will not. You're just like your father. Hit first and listen later. I won't let you hit Jimmy.

JIMMY (Persecutor): I love you, Mommy. Why does Daddy like to beat me?

Sarah switched to rescuing Jimmy. Then Kip switched to persecuting Sarah and she responded by putting Kip in the found-out villain's role of Victim. Little Jimmy intuitively knew the play and switched to persecuting Kip with a plaintive, "Why does Daddy like to beat me?" Jimmy then sat back in his Little Professor and watched the new Drama, "Let Mommy and Daddy fight."

We play all the roles at one time or another but have one

favorite role which we assume more often. Although a few players consciously set up the Drama and select their parts, role assumption is usually an unconscious act from the Parent or Child. The recordings in our head, family patterns, and experiences direct us toward the roles which will meet our stroking needs. Each time we take on a role, we are making another payment on the mortgage.

Victim

Fat fever sufferers operate from a Victim role.
- I'm too fat be handsome.
- Joe got the brains and I got the fat.
- Every time I diet, something happens to disrupt it.
- My weight is hereditary; there is no way out, I'm stuck with it.
- I'm fat and my two lucky sisters are slender.
- Someone has to be fat, but why me?

Fat people feel victimized for the following reasons:
- They are put down constantly.
- They have fewer friends.
- They are less attractive to the opposite sex.
- They have fewer meaningful social encounters.
- They are less successful at work.
- They lack the energy for a full and active life.
- They are more susceptible to disease.
- They die sooner.
- They are the butt of jokes and crooked humor.
- They even pay to be fat: excessive eating increases food costs, insurance rates, the cost of clothes, and medication and drug costs as well as causing a higher rate of absenteeism at work and in some cases even requiring specially sized furniture and equipment.

Discounts

The Victim role assumed by fat fever sufferers is stimulated by "discounts." The obese people of our society have a great deal of difficulty accepting a compliment. Obese people are so used to being put down by verbal or nonverbal cold or zigzag strokes that they usually discount warm strokes by a statement which reduces the stroking value.

GEORGE (warm stroke): That's a pretty dress, Sally.

SALLY (discount): I bet you see it more like a camouflage net than a dress.

PETER (warm stroke): Gerry, we feel that your personality would be effective in customer services. Would you like to try it for a while?

GERRY (discount): O.K., if you don't mind a blimp on the front counter.

PAULA (warm stroke): Jean, I'm pleased you were elected as our representative; congratulations.

JEAN (discount): It's really nothing. I don't think anyone else wanted the job. Most of the girls have too full a social life to spare the time.

Discounting becomes so ingrained in a fat person's behavior that it is continued even after the excess weight is lost. It is not unusual to observe a once-fat person who discounts each warm stroke as if he or she were still obese. The person who is successful in losing weight may continue feeling victimized until he or she learns to "think thin." I will always remember a young man saying to his sister who had lost 40 pounds: "Look in the mirror—you're beautiful. You've got all my friends drooling. Why do you still think fat?"

EXERCISE: HOW DO I DISCOUNT? LET US COUNT THE WAYS.

1. Make a list of ways in which you discount strokes.

2. What action can you take now to eliminate discounting?

3. In column 1, make a list of ten words or phrases which indicate you "think fat." In column 2, change to words or phrases which say "think thin."

	1 "Think Fat" Words	2 "Think Thin" Words
1		
2		
3		
4		
5		
6		
7		
8		
9		
10		

Make a decision now to use the "think thin" terminology.

Injunctions

Fat fever sufferers are restrained from a continuing cure by a number of "injunctions" which are programmed or which they decided to adopt when they were young children. An injunction, in the simplest terms, is a message which starts with a "don't."

Some injunctions which stimulate fat fever and prohibit, decrease the likelihood of, or postpone a cure are:

• "Don't be slim." This injunction is transmitted to boys by parental figures who relate fatness to health and size and weight to manliness. Some parents use this injunction on daughters as a chastity belt: the boys won't like her and she'll stay with me if she remains fat. Parents who feel this way about a daughter, usually have a hang-up about their own behavior or the behavior of some other family member. Somewhere in the murky past there may be a "Goldilocks" who jumped from bed to bed, or Father may be concerned about his own sexual urges and fear of incest.

• "Don't act." This injunction is transmitted to obese people by parental figures who say it is O.K. to be fat. "Don't diet, you'll grow out of fatness," "Don't diet, you'll only become ill." The obese person who accepts this injunction often received parental strokes for fatness. Although they may half-heartedly try a diet, they usually regress to passivity about weight control as a means to attract similar, parental strokes.

• "Don't think." This injunction is transmitted to obese people by parental figures who say, "Don't waste your time looking for a nonexistent cure—everyone in our family is fat. Don't use transactional analysis to identify your program—it's only another fad. Don't find a cure or I'll have to recognize my own weakness."

• "Don't feel." This injunction is transmitted to obese people by parental figures who say, "Don't feel bad because the other children tease you. Don't feel hurt because you're not asked to the party—who cares about an old party anyway? Don't feel bad because you are never chosen for a team—being the referee is even better."

• "Don't do anything; you may get hurt or ill. Don't climb the wall. 'Humpty Dumpty fell off a wall and all the king's horses and all the king's men couldn't put Humpty Dumpty together again.' " The obese person with this injunction may spend a lifetime putting off the decision to cure fat fever.

EXERCISE: MY DON'TS

1. Describe three injunctions [2] which are restraining you from curing fat fever. You made the decision during childhood to accept these injunctions and to continue activating them in later life. You can also make the decision to eliminate, defuse, or deactivate these injunctions. List ways to deal with your don'ts.

My Don'ts	How to Deal with My Don'ts
A.	
B.	
C.	

Persecutor

The Persecutor role is attributed to the luck of the draw, heredity, society, friends, family, and the good life, glands, and other illnesses.

· Dad and Mom are both heavy—so no wonder.
· My boyfriend loves to eat and he tempts me.
· Sally pushes food on me constantly.
· I could lose weight if I didn't have these glands.
· The availability of food and drink around here disrupts every diet I try.

There is a vast difference between being persecuted and being influenced. We are indeed programmed for obesity by our family pattern; heredity accounts for some physical characteristics; the abundance of the good life and the influence of friends and family stimulate eating and drinking. These are influences only. You are your own fat fever Persecutor. You are responsible for being fat. You are fat because you choose to be fat. A cure is only possible when you accept the fact that no one else is persecuting you.

Rescuer

There is no point in searching for a Rescuer.

• Your physician can prescribe a diet but you alone can execute the order.

• A weight-control organization, club, or group can provide advice and support but only you can activate the program.

• A health club can provide an exercise plan but only you can decide to participate.

• This book can provide insight into your program and separate symptoms and causes but only you can decide to work through the exercises thoroughly and use the outputs.

Fat fever is a tragic and personally destructive Drama in which the performer may play all three roles. The fat fever Victim is also the real Persecutor and must cancel the play's run. The search for a Parent or Child Rescuer must be replaced by the fat fever sufferer playing an Adult role based on analysis of background data, a planned cure, and a personal contract to execute the plan. The rational, logical Adult problem solver is a factual nonfeeling state and replaces the feeling-state Parent or Child Rescuer. The Adult discards the unsupported Persecutor reactions of blaming and criticizing others and the inappropriate Victim reactions of helplessness and giving up. The Adult bases cure planning on reality, not feelings.

EXERCISE: MY DRAMAS

1. Describe one food- or weight-related Drama in which you were involved.

2. How did you feel after the Drama? Did you enjoy or dislike the role(s)?

3. What Adult behaviors can you use to reduce Dramas and role assumption?

FAT FEVER POSITIONS

There are four classifications of "life positions."

I'm not O.K.—You're O.K.	Unconscious feeling
I'm not O.K.—You're not O.K.	Unconscious feeling
I'm O.K.—You're not O.K.	Unconscious feeling
I'm O.K.—You're O.K.	Conscious position

Early on, a child may accept the I'm not O.K.—You're O.K. position. If this position is not confirmed, within a few years, the child settles on the I'm not O.K.—You're not O.K. or I'm O.K.—You're not O.K. This position remains part of the person's existence for the rest of his or her life unless there is an Adult decision to change to I'm O.K.—You're O.K.[3]

Fat people have considerable difficulty and internal turmoil over settling on one life position. The very different responses to eating, weight, and Kitchen behavior from social interactions create intense fluctuations in how the obese person views his or her O.K.-ness. An obese person who makes an Adult conclusion in favor of the I'm O.K.—You're O.K. position is as rare as hen's teeth.

The I'm not O.K.–You're O.K. position says my experience and feelings tell me that I am a powerless Child/Victim. You have all the power and will persecute me, rescue me or leave me alone depending on whether you are in the Helping or Controlling Parent.

When obese people gather together because they are fat, they are perpetuating the I'm not O.K–You're not O.K. position. We can't do anything about our weight, so we'll keep away from the O.K. people. We'll sit around, cry, moan, complain, and commiserate with each other as we pile on more pounds in this "let's die" position.

The I'm O.K.–You're not O.K. position says my experience and feelings tell me that I am the power Parent and you are the powerless Child/Victim. When I am in the Helping Parent I'll be your Rescuer, but when I am in the Controlling Parent I'll be your Persecutor. I may decide to leave you to flounder alone or get rid of you in one way or another.

The I'm O.K.–You're O.K. position says my Adult concludes that we can get on with doing and living. Everything is not perfect but we can cope mutually with the issues. It is the "Let's Live a Full Life" position.

Although a baby is unfettered at birth, the early feeling of a Kitchen-developing child is I'm not O.K.–You're O.K. The big people force food on the little people who do not have the physical power to rebel. The child pushes the bottle away, bites the teat, or spits out the strained mush only to have it forced back. The child has no recourse but to adapt to the forced feeding and then lie around with cramps.

Little people feel that the big people are O.K. but they are Not O.K. Little people realize that big people can force them to eat, make them uncomfortable, punish them by yelling or even inflicting physical pain. When they eat up, they avoid unpleasantness and get some needed strokes even if it is only through the burping ritual.

Eventually, when such a little person has gained a little strength, rebellion against eating becomes normal behavior. The primary Kitchen-oriented person meets the rebellion head-on with force and punishment. The young person is checking out the position and by losing once again reinforces the I'm not O.K.—You're O.K. feeling.

Some children are experts at "pig-trough warfare." They seem to pick the right time and place to rebel and know what behavior will have the most impact on Mommy and Daddy. When Mommy gives up or cries in frustration, little Joey has feedback which says, "Maybe I'm not O.K.—but I feel a little more O.K. now and you're not O.K. when I win the battle." One young mother, involved in "pig-trough warfare," commented, "I know he's had enough when either one of us starts to cry."

The young developing Kitchen person receives a stream of messages which make him or her think it's O.K. to be overweight.
 • You're a chip off the old block.
 • Boy, is he ever sturdy!
 • Those few extra pounds will help her during the flu season.
 • My future football star is built like a tank.
 • Here, I'll rub your cute round tummy.
This O.K.-ness about weight is reinforced when the little person goes out to play. Heavy children use their weight to intimidate their more slender playmates. Shoving or knocking Paul down until he cries provides input which says: "I'm stronger"; "He's a crybaby"; "I'm the boss; I can punish Paul just like Daddy punishes me." The little person is saying, "Right now I'm O.K. and Paul is not O.K."

Recently, I observed a grossly overweight boy using his bulk to knock down two other boys at every opportunity. My first Parent reaction was "what a bully." It turned out that they were playing "Cannon," based on a television crime program. The fat boy was the hero, Cannon, and the other boys were the bad guys. It will be a traumatic moment for this fat boy when he has to face up to the fact that "Cannon" is fiction, not reality.

Cannon's popularity may be due to the desire of 70 million

obese people for a hero to whom they can relate. Cannon may be reinforcing the message that it's O.K. to be fat in much the same way that Kojak implies that baldness is a sign of virility.

When obese children attend school, they find out that being fat may be O.K. at home but is a "no-no" at school. Teachers and classmates transmit a continual stream of messages and put-downs which say, "I'm O.K., but you, Fatty, are not O.K."

- Johnny, we'll have to do something about your weight.
- The skim milk is for Johnny.
- Children, why should Johnny stop eating candy?
- Yes, it will ruin his teeth, but I was thinking of something else. Mary, it is not nice to call people fat slobs even if your father does it. See, you've hurt Johnny's feelings.
- But I don't want to dance with Johnny. He dances like an elephant.
- Johnny, you can't be on our team. You run too slowly and besides, my Daddy says fatties stink when they sweat.
- Fat Johnny Jones can't feel his bones.

Early school days are traumatic for obese children who start out with a Kitchen message that being a "chip off the old block" is O.K. but soon find out that it is not O.K. to be a "stave off the old barrel." Children, especially in groups, are extremely cruel and are quick to tease and pick on a fat child.

Some insensitive teachers pass out not-O.K. signals about weight by direct comments or by body language. Jill said, "I hate my health class. When Mrs. Mayne talks about the kinds of food we should eat and how much, she stares at me."

Obese children find it difficult if not impossible to gain acceptance from average-weight classmates. It is not by choice that not-O.K. fat kids join not-O.K. fat friends.

Parents who program Johnny for obesity are throwing him into the lion's den. These parents rationalize Johnny's dislike of school but seldom face up to their responsibility. Children may be cruel antagonists but the parent who created fat Johnny is infinitely more cruel and destructive.

On occasion, one child in a Kitchen family will remain

slender as the remainder of the family piles on the pounds. Parental warm strokes are provided to obese children for being chips off the old block. The slender child becomes aware of the differences and the not-O.K. feelings are reinforced by cold stroke put-downs—"I don't know what to do with you; you're thin as a rail, all skin and bones"—or by ridiculing names like Billy Bones, Sammy Skeleton, and Tommy Toothpick. School days are traumatic as the slender child finds out that being thin is O.K. and the obese child learns that obesity is a not-O.K. condition. Jason said, "I really felt bad for my twin, Jack. Mom and Dad were pleased that he was healthy and let me know that I was the thin, ugly duckling. The tables turned when we went to school. School was hell for Jack. The kids tormented him and called him 'Jumbo Jackie.' I tried to protect and comfort Jackie because I knew what it was like to be put down. Our parents sure sold us a bill of goods. In my early years, I wanted to gain weight to be O.K. and all of a sudden Jack had to lose weight to be O.K. We were programmed to be twin losers."

The I'm not O.K.—you're O.K. feelings are accentuated during the young adult years. Obese persons are less social and receive fewer party invitations, are less active and athletic, and are less attractive to the opposite sex. Their choice is to continue being lonely or to do something about their obesity. In some cases, especially among females, the mating ritual stimulates weight reduction. Losing weight at this time does not mean achieving an I'm-O.K. feeling. The person may feel a bit better but it is a plastic feeling as the weight is regained after the mating dance is successful.

Case

Sara had 170 pounds on a 5-foot-2-inch frame at 17 years of age. Eventually, the mating ritual stimulated her to starve herself until she reached 120 pounds. A vivacious, beautiful woman had been lurking behind the blubber. Even though the weight was gone, she still felt not O.K. She worried continuously about what other people thought of her and reacted with despair at each weight fluctuation. It was readily apparent that after the mating ritual she would pile on the pounds. Losing weight does not make a person feel O.K. unless the person deals with the internal messages. Sara failed because at 120 pounds she continued to think fat.

Persons who remain obese or gain weight during later years continue to receive not-O.K. signals.

• Fat Molly slaves in the stuffy back room while pretty Rose serves the customers.

• Fat Jack taught the last three supervisors the job but is not considered managerial material.

• Fat Carol turns hopefully at every whistle, only to find the approving stares on slender Mary.

• Fat Ned never gets visibility by training executives. Slim Jim does that while Fat Ned trains the foremen.

• Fat Gracie sits alone night after night waiting for Ed to come home. He, of course, is out with the boys—or is he?

• Fat Freddy is shattered when curvy Cindy runs away with terrific Tom.

Some obese people, who have been programmed strictly, continue to operate from an I'm O.K.—You're not O.K. position. Blaming others, making excuses, and originating Hurt activities are usual ways to reinforce this position. These people are nearly impossible to work, live, or socialize with because they do not take any responsibility for their behavior. It is always someone else's fault.

• She wriggled into the job on her back.

• He must be related to the boss.

• It's your fault that I can't lose weight.

• The doctor gave me a stupid diet; it doesn't work.

• Overweight people perform just as well as average-weight people, if not better, but our company has a secret policy on promotion.

• I miss a few days here and there for sickness, but it's not my fault that I have fallen arches. Why should I be penalized?

A fat fever cure is only possible when the sufferer makes a

rational and logical Adult decision to change to an I'm O.K.–You're O.K. position. This means not only maintaining an average, healthy weight but removing the internal recordings which say "think fat." I'm O.K.–You're O.K. people trust and like themselves, provide legitimate strokes, receive strokes graciously without discounting their worth, and are open and leveling but sensitive to the feelings of others.

Progress to the cure position I'm O.K.–Your're O.K. is possible only when fat fever sufferers trust themselves sufficiently to disclose the early recordings which support their feelings about the noncure positions I'm not O.K.–You're O.K., I'm not O.K.–You're not O.K., I'm O.K.–You're not O.K. Disclosed feelings and actions are related or compared to the present behaviors which perpetuate fat fever. Knowing how a feeling or behavior originated not only assists but is a necessity for corrective action.

Curing fat fever is not an easy task which can be done instantly. It took years to assimilate and refine the Kitchen program and it will take time to reprogram. The time involved is different for each person, depending on how badly the person wants to change and how much the person trusts himself or herself to live and cope with the change. Taking the medicine is not pleasant but reaching the understanding and eventual success which form the cure provides a feeling of euphoria which makes it all worthwhile

EXERCISE: FAT FEVER POSITIONS

1. Consider each element carefully and decide on a word or phrase which describes your feeling about the element. Write your response in the life-position column which best fits your feeling.

Elements	1 I'm not O.K. You're O.K.	2 I'm not O.K. You're Not O.K.	3 I'm O.K. You're Not O.K.	4 I'm O.K. You're O.K.
Family				
Home				
Work				
Community				
Education				
Friends				
Social life				
Recreation				
Affection				
Ambition				
Promotion				
Change				
Conflict				
Obesity				

2. The entries above indicate your life position. Do you wish to change? If so, what can you do to facilitate an orderly change?

RACKET BUSTING

Each person is capable of many different feelings. Some feelings, such as loneliness when a loved one passes away, are legitimate, while other feelings are acted out, phony parts in the person's program. Parental messages, originated in the Kitchen, Bathroom, Hurt, and Love family patterns, are reinforced repeatedly until the Adapted Child accepts them as reality. The parental messages—which continuously tell a child "You are stupid," "You are clever," "You are hateful," or "You are spiteful"—tattoo a recurring feeling in the subconscious which the person displays regularly through life. These favorite recurring feelings are called rackets.[4]

When you observe friends, relatives, co-workers, customers, neighbors, or other acquaintances who are always:

- Guilty
- Frustrated
- Sad
- Fearful
- Hungry
- Envious
- Hateful
- Inadequate
- Resentful
- Suspicious

you are observing a racket in operation.

Rackets develop from Controlling Parent (CP) and Helpful Parent (HP) messages, originated in a family pattern, accepted in the Adapted Child (AC), and played out in a drama role.

HP and CP Messages	Pattern	AC Racket	Role
CP Always get in the first blow.	Hurt	Hurt	Persecutor
HP Always help the underdog.	Love	Help	Rescuer
HP Turn the other cheek.	Love	Forgive	Rescuer
CP Always eat "three squares" a day.	Kitchen	Hunger	Victim
CP Eat up or else—Pow!!	Kitchen	Fear	Victim
CP Your pimples and blackheads are repulsive.	Bathroom	Shame	Victim
CP When will you ever learn toilet training. You must be stupid or lazy.	Bathroom	Inadequacy	Victim

Parental messages about eating habits, food, and weight, which are communicated regularly to young children, may initiate a variety of destructive fat-fever-producing rackets. Some examples are:

- Providing sweets as a reward may initiate a craving racket.
- Using food as a punishment may initiate a threatened racket.
- Feeding by force may initiate a fear racket.
- Stroking for being overweight may initiate a false-pride or vanity racket.
- Controlling others by using weight may initiate a bully racket.
- Saying eating solves every physical or emotional problems may initiate a hunger racket.
- Using weight as a put-down may initiate a shame racket.
- Forcing a child to sit until unwanted food is finished may initiate a slowpoke or procrastination racket.
- Providing special food, such as ice cream, when a child is ill may initiate a malingering racket.
- Stroking for "eating up" may initiate a gluttony racket.
- Comparing eating habits may initiate a guilt racket.

Although the recurring feeling is executed in a variety of ways, obese or potentially obese persons can often trace their rackets to programming related to food or weight. Cure requires removal of these rackets.

Racket busting is an Adult problem-solving activity. Identification of the racket is relatively simple but upsetting. The realization that many of the times we were ashamed, guilty, envious, or experienced some other recurrent feeling were based on prejudicial parental messages can be a shock.

Case

Gerry was ashamed and resentful about his weight. When his feelings became too much to bear, he turned for relief to the bottle. This led to periods of hatefulness and aggression toward family, friends, and co-workers. Gerry's excuse was, "I'm in one of my moods. I don't know why I feel this way, so just keep out of my path. It'll pass in a few days." During a study group, Gerry said, "When I was small my mother said 'Eat up' and Dad said 'It's O.K. to be built like a truck.' At school I found out that I was a not-O.K. dump truck. Winning by using my weight became less and less possible until I was losing most of the time. In high school, I was ashamed to be fat and guilty that I was unable to lose weight. When I went to work, I found out that physical appearance had more influence on progress than productivity. Fat people never get the good jobs in our shop. Now I know what my racket is, and although I haven't erased it completely, I have it under control. When I feel my resentful racket surfacing, I say, "No—not today. I'm going to feel O.K., not lousy. I don't have to be resentful because I can cope now. I still drink, but for enjoyment, not as a release. The big difference is that I haven't been smashed or fought with Sally for weeks."

EXERCISE: WHAT IS MY RACKET?

Racket identification comes from self-analysis:

1. What feelings do you have which seem to smother you time and time again? Identify one primary feeling (recurring most often) and one secondary feeling (recurring less often).

2. Do you ever say, "I don't know why I feel this way—it's only one of my moods"?

3. Do you enjoy your recurring feelings?

4. We tend to structure our lives to reexperience old and favored feelings. How do you set up the drama for your racket?

5. Has anyone ever asked you why you are always so hateful, miserable, unhappy, resentful, grouchy, hostile, etc.? How would you answer this question for your own racket?

6. Recall and describe how your primary and secondary rackets were programmed.

Primary:

Secondary:

7. What Adult action can you take to bust your racket(s)?

STAMPING OUT FAT FEVER

Have you ever felt hurt by, annoyed at, or insulted by another person without reacting immediately? Later on, did you repay that person with a curt remark or a put-down? Have you ever awaited your chance to make a protagonist look stupid, clumsy, or inadequate? If so, you have collected a feeling, stored it away in your memory, and cashed it in when you were ready.

Trading in psychological "stamps" is the transactional analysis description for dealing with these collected feelings.[5] The term is borrowed from the retailers who provide stamps, with each purchase, which are stored in books and eventually traded in for prizes ranging from a toothbrush to a trip around the world.

Although each retailer has different-colored stamps and different stamp values for each prize, the lists of prizes are similar. The collector makes the decision on which retailer's stamps to collect, what prize to strive for, and when to cash in or trade the stamps. Some stamp collectors set their sights on a major prize (automobile, boat, trailer) while others cash in more often for lesser prizes (coffee pot, barbecue, picnic hamper). Although the objective may be a major prize, it is not unusual for frustrated stamp collectors to change their minds and cash in for a lesser payoff.

People deal in feelings in a similar way. We decide what feelings or stamps to collect, how long to keep them, and how and for what payoff the feelings will be traded. Some people retain their stamp collections until they have enough for a major prize (assault, rape, murder) while others are content with cashing them in more often for lesser prizes (put-downs, insults, absenteeism, intoxication).

Each stamp collected adds to frustration, resentment, and discontent (like a "slow burn") until a payoff is needed. When someone says, "I worked like hell today, I'm going to have a third piece of pie," that person is trading in the resentment about working hard as justification for eating excessively.

We structure our activities and manipulate others in ways that allow us to reexperience our rackets and to fill our stamp books. When we have collected enough good stamps, we cash them in by doing something for ourselves. When we have collected enough bad stamps, we cash them in by doing something to someone else.

Just as we have favorite rackets and an unconscious life position, we have favorite-colored stamps.

- Brown stamps represent bad feelings generally.
- Gold stamps represent good feelings generally.
- Red stamps represent anger/hostility.
- Green stamps represent envy.
- Blue stamps represent sadness/pessimism.
- White stamps represent purity.

- Yellow stamps represent fear/cowardliness.
- Black stamps represent feelings of being overwhelmed/depression.
  - Silver stamps represent hope/optimism.
  - Pink stamps represent happiness.
  - Violet stamps represent serenity.

Stamps may be cashed in immediately or stored for shorter or longer periods of time. Once a stamp is collected, it will be cashed in eventually unless the collector makes an Adult decision to discard the stamp.

Example

In the fall of 1941, I had just purchased my first automobile, a 1928 4-cylinder Chrysler, for $60 ($8 down and $2 a week with no interest payments). One day my friend Bob and I decided to paint "Old Chrys" with the green and black paint which he had scrounged from his father. The painting took longer than expected and we worked long into the night to finish underneath the corner streetlight.

The next day was Saturday and I drove proudly over to pick up Bob at work. While I was waiting at a red light, Jack and another member of a rival baseball team doubled up with laughter as they inspected my sparkling new paint job. As I started away, Jack yelled out, "Laverty, you dumb bastard, your old crate is covered with bugs." As soon as I got out of their sight, I stopped to find out what he meant. I was shattered. The back of "Old Chrys" was covered with moths, flies, mosquitoes, and other insects which had been attracted by the street light and stuck in the wet paint.

In 1952, Jack reported into an army unit where I was the transport officer. I directed the transport sergeant to put Jack on fuel tankers instead of in the staff car pool, reasoning that he was too mouthy for staff car duty. Here it was 11 years later and I had cashed my brown stamp by assigning Jack to the dirtiest job in the transport pool.

Fat fever sufferers trade in a wide range of bad-feeling stamps. Many brown-stamp collectors cash in on some other person, but fat people have a tendency to cash in on themselves. Although they may feel that they are indulging their Child by their cashing activities, in reality they are often persecuting themselves, fat fever Victims.

Case

YELLOW STAMPS.

Nora was 70 pounds overweight and had faced years of frustrating, unsuccessful dieting. She had a collection of yellow fear stamps. Nora was born 3 months after her father's death, which resulted in her forming a very close relationship with her mother. Nora was afraid and worried constantly about the day her mother would die. She was sure that without her mother's comfort and support she would go insane. Nora structured her activities to reinforce her need to collect yellow stamps and even went so far as to check carefully the ages of persons listed in newspaper obituary columns. She became very frightened and depressed each time an acquaintance of her mother's age died. Nora traded her yellow stamps for excessive amounts of food as her Parent said, "You will feel better after you eat."

Nora is changing her life position I'm not O.K.—You're O.K. to I'm O.K.—You're O.K. She is learning about her stamp collection and developing internal signals to stop collecting yellow stamps. For the first time, she is losing weight and is in a "Let's Live" position.

GREEN STAMPS.

Obese people envy the "beautiful people." They daydream and night dream about what it would be like to be muscular like Paul, wear a bikini like Denise, wear glamorous clothes like Martha, or even be whistled at, just once. Green-stamp collections are traded for isolation, such as keeping away from the beautiful people and reducing recreational, social, and physical activities to situations where there is no competition and lots of food.

RED STAMPS.

Obese people collect red anger stamps. They are constantly angry internally and externally about their inability to lose weight. They blame others for their eating habits, the doctor for an unworkable diet, and the system for restricting their progress. They cash their red stamps in on eating, drinking, violence, or uproar. The fat person who curses, yells, breaks furniture, or assaults others is cashing in red stamps.

BLUE STAMPS.

I have yet to meet a fat person who does not collect blue sad stamps. They are sad and unhappy about their shape, size, work life, social life, family life, and general physical and psychological condition. Some fat people make a valiant effort to trade their sad feelings for the "jolly fatman" routine. When obese people masquerade behind self-deprecating humor, they are cashing their stamps in on themselves. Although it may appear an O.K. activity on the surface, fat people trying the false-humor routine are increasing their sad stamps. Each time a fat man puts himself down, he is collecting a sad feeling.

Case

During one study-group meeting, Tony was asked why he was always pleasant. He gave the stock fat man's reply, "I can't fight or run so it's safer to be pleasant." Another participant asked, "Are you really happy?" Tony replied, "Hell no, no fat person is really happy. Underneath it all, I am the saddest of the sad. I guess I have been wearing a clown's costume to hide my true feelings."

Later on, Tony mentioned that this was the first time he had been honest about his feelings. He was collecting blue stamps and cashing them in by putting himself down, which was increasing rather than decreasing his collection.

The phony activity of personal put-downs, in the name of humor, is very harmful. The fat man who thinks people are laughing with him is mistaken. There is a big difference between laughing with a person and laughing at a person. Most people laugh at, not with, fatties.

It is impossible to reduce or stop collecting blue stamps while indulging in destructive put-downs. Obese people must face reality: fatness is nothing to joke about; fat people do not have to entertain at their own expense; playing the clown is O.K. in the circus but inappropriate in real life. When a fat man is the target for his own jokes, he is saying:

• "I'm not O.K.–You're O.K., so I'll play the not-O.K. clown. Laugh at me so that I can fill up my stamp collection. Later I'll be able to trade my stamps in for 12 beers and a large pizza with double pepperoni."

• "It's sure nice to have good friends who are ready and willing to laugh at my misfortune. I don't know how I would propel myself on a self-destructive course, if it weren't for your laughter. Thanks for the gallows transaction."

It is not easy for an individual who has played the clown for years to drop the destructive habit. Awareness of the phoniness of the activity helps reduce the frequency of "fat humor." Recalling "fat humor" incidents and analyzing the situation, cause, outcome, and feelings are helpful also. It is important that persons seeking a fat-fever-cure contract with themselves to jump off the fat humor wagon.

It is not easy to get off the fat humor wagon. Occupying center stage and attracting laughter (no matter how phony) is like a drug to some people. If your Child is hooked in this way, change the subject matter of your jokes from "how fat I am" to "how amusing life is" or some other planned script. You will still get laughs but not at your own expense.

BLACK STAMPS. Most sufferers are overwhelmed by fat fever. Trying and crying year after year, diet after diet, hurt after hurt, is a give-up feeling. When the stamp collection turns black, the sufferer is crying, "What's the use? There's no way out. I've tried and tried but I can't do it. I'm not O.K., I'll stay fat until the day I die and the sooner I die the better off I'll be."

Black stamps indicate that obese persons are at the end of

their rope. They have tried everything. Their life is coming apart around them. Social life is almost nonexistent. Family breakdown is happening. Work is drudgery. A large black-stamp collection is a prelude to serious physical and emotional illness.

Case

Five years after her marriage to Max, Dianne had changed from a 125-pound sexpot to a less appealing 180 pounder. Max tried to help her cope and take responsibility for her condition, but Dianne blamed childbirth as the culprit even though there was no medical evidence to substantiate her claim.

Dianne gathered a variety of brown stamps and traded them in for more food. Max refused to go out with her and she became, for all intents and purposes isolated behind four walls. Eventually, she would not even do the weekly grocery shopping. Max was also collecting brown stamps and trading them in for nights out and one affair after another. Eventually, Max left to live with a 125-pound sexpot.

Dianne's stamp collection turned black. At 28 she had lost her husband, had no friends, and had acquired a 3-year-old daughter. Her family, who lived in another city, would have welcomed her home but Dianne could not face them. When in her teens she had lost 40 pounds she had bragged to her fat sister that weight would never be a problem again.

Dianne admitted that she was so overwhelmed by her black-stamp collection that she had contemplated self-destruction. During one black period, she turned on the gas stove but came to her senses when she heard her child crying. Dianne made a contract to stop blaming from the Controlling Parent and to stop indulging her Adapted Child. By taking responsibility for her condition and making an Adult decision to cure it, Dianne has discarded her black stamps and initiated her own cure. She feels more O.K. now than she has for years and is planning a "Let's Live" position.

GOLD STAMPS. Obese people seldom collect gold good-feeling stamps. Gold stamps say: "I've done a good job; I'm successful;

I'm acceptable; I look good; generally I appreciate myself; all things considered, I'm O.K."

Few people develop the inner strength which allows them to do without gold stamps—self-appreciation. Although the ideal would be to eliminate all stamp collections, the ideal is not possible. We all need a few gold, pink, or violet stamps to trade in when we need a lift.

The most rational strategy for curing fat fever is to replace the brown bad-feeling stamps with gold good-feeling stamps. As sufferers progress to an appropriate healthy weight, they collect good feelings which they can trade for warm strokes and other forms of positive reinforcement. Reaching a condition-category milestone is a good feeling which is traded for a reward.

Changing to a gold stamp collection can be done best by learning how to accept warm strokes graciously. This means accepting warm strokes without the usual discounts which are so common from fat people.

JAMIE (warm stroke): Myrtle, you sure look good. I'm proud to take you out.

MYRTLE (discount): Come on, I don't look all that good. I'm still 16 pounds overweight.

MYRTLE (gracious acceptance): Thanks, Jamie. I'm glad you're pleased. We'll have a good time together.

Once a fat fever cure is stabilized and the person has made a conscious change to an I'm O.K.—You're O.K. position, Adult action is initiated to reduce the gold-stamp collection. The I'm O.K.—You're O.K. person is sufficiently comfortable within to get along with a minimum stamp collection. The independent feeling of knowing you are in complete control and that you will remain in control of your mind and body is enough for most O.K. people.

EXERCISE: STAMP COLLECTION

1. Family patterns influence children to collect and trade in specific feelings. One may say that a child is programmed to feel in a certain way.

 • Kitchen people trade in their feelings for food-related

payoffs. Their slogan is Food Cures Everything.

• Bathroom people trade in their feelings for body-waste-related payoffs. Their slogan is Bowel Movements Cure Everything.

• Hurt people trade in their feelings for hostility-related payoffs. Their slogan is Strike Out.

• Love people trade in their feelings for affection-related payoffs. Their slogan is We Speak Kindness Here.

On the following table, describe a specific example of how you collect and trade in brown stamps. Did this feeling originate in Kitchen, Bathroom, Hurt or Love patterns?

Stamp-Collection Example	Trading Prize	Origin: Kitchen, Bathroom Hurt, Love
Red (anger) stamp:		
Green (envy) stamp:		
Blue (sad) stamp:		
White (purity) stamp:		
Yellow (fear) stamp:		
Black (depression) stamp:		
Other brown (bad-feeling) stamps:		

2. How does the prize/payoff for your stamps influence fat fever?

3. List two Adult decisions which you can make to reduce your brown-stamp collection.

A.

B.

7

Fat Fever Games

People play hundreds of psychological games.[1] The games described here are those which initiate, reinforce, and advance fat fever.

The elements of a psychological game are:

1. Two or more persons play the roles of Persecutor, Rescuer, and Victim.

2. One person initiates the game from a Persecutor or Victim role. This is an invitation to others to join the game.

3. Communication between players appear to be No Surprise—legitimate transactions.

4. The reason for the game is obscured by a Hidden transaction.

5. The game ends with a negative payoff where one or more players are physically or emotionally hurt.

We are programmed to play certain games much as we are programmed in ego states, family patterns, rackets, stamps, and life positions. Our programming leads us to participate in a favorite recurring game with only the time, setting, and characters changing. The game may be a casual encounter with a minor negative payoff (put-downs, avoidance, rejection) or a critical encounter with a major negative payoff (termination of employment, assault, death).

Games are played to pass time, to attract strokes, and to reexperience old favorite feelings. Games, strategies, tactics, moves, and payoffs are unlimited. Almost every day new games or new switches to old games are identified. The games described here are related directly to fat fever.

"Chastity Belt"

The game of "Chastity Belt" ("Chastity Jock") is initiated by I'm-not-O.K. persons with inadequacy, insecurity, or fear rackets. They worry constantly that their handsome or beautiful mate will leave them or be attracted away by another handsome or beautiful person.

The not-O.K. spouse can be recognized by statements such as:

• You're so beautiful. I often wonder what you see in me. (Inadequacy racket)

• You're so handsome. I'm jealous when other women look at you. (Insecurity racket)

• I don't like crowds or dancing. Let's stay home so that we can be alone. (Fear racket)

• No wife of mine will wear a bikini or low-cut gown. (Purity racket)

The not-O.K. spouse is playing back internal mistrust and fear messages.

• Sally's beautiful; I've got to keep my eye on her.

• I'd better meet him after the office party.

• I'll have to do something about that good-looking secretary.

• Her clothes are too revealing (or youthful) for a mother of two.

• I'll meet him on Fridays because that is the action day.

"Chastity Belt" is a variation on the old strategy, "Keep her pregnant, barefoot, and in the kitchen." The not-O.K. person initiates the game from the Little Professor/Persecutor by pushing and even forcing excessive food, mainly of the high-calorie variety, on an unsuspecting mate who is expected to receive the "eat more" message in the Adapted Child/Victim role. Although the initiating role is persecutor, the not-O.K. spouse pretends that he or she is the Helping Parent/Rescuer or Adapted Child/Victim in the drama.

PRETEND RESCUER: A little more stew won't hurt you. You work hard. Anyway, a few more pounds will make you even more attractive.

PRETEND VICTIM: I cooked all day to surprise you and now you don't want a second helping. Have a little more to show that you appreciate my cooking.

The Persecutor's reasoning for initiating "Chastity Belt" is:

• Fat people are less attractive.

• A chastity belt made of fat, with me keeping the key, means protection and security.

• Fatness binds a marriage together.

• Fat people have less choice and less opportunity to be unfaithful.

The potential Victim can comply in the Adapted Child by eating, by gaining weight, and by generally going to pot. The Persecutor may feel more secure, but the Victim must adapt to a lifetime of fat misery.

Some insecure parents initiate "Chastity Belt" with their children. The parents who live in fear of the shame of an umarried, pregnant daughter may resort to encircling her with a chastity belt of fat. Other parents use the game to restrict their offspring's social opportunities and thereby keep the young birds in the nest.

The potential Victim can refuse to play the game. This is done by a Surprise transaction which lets the Persecutor know that the game is called because the intended Victim has moved from stomach to brain. The Persecutor may continue to manipulate from the Little Professor or switch to the Controlling Parent to force compliance. The potential Victim deals with this force by replying continually from the logical, rational Adult. Surprise responses will cross the transaction, create some tension, and possibly initiate an argument or fight, but this is more acceptable than succumbing to fat fever.

ILLUSTRATION 16: HOOKED CHILD JOINS THE GAME

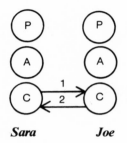

1. SARA (Little Professor/Persecutor):
Come on, dear, have a second piece of shortcake.

2. JOE (Adapted Child/Victim):
O.K., I love shortcake.

ILLUSTRATION 17: REFUSING TO PLAY

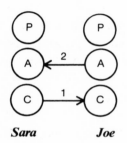

1. SARA (Little Professor/Persecutor):
Come on, dear, have a second piece of shortcake.

2. JOE (Adult):
No thanks, I'm watching my diet.

ILLUSTRATION 18: PERSECUTOR'S SWITCH TO CONTROLLING PARENT

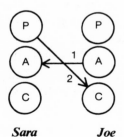

1. JOE (Adult):
No thanks, I'm watching my diet.

2. SARA (Controlling Parent/Persecutor):
You don't need to diet. Now eat up and don't be so silly.

ILLUSTRATION 19: PERSECUTOR'S SWITCH TO ADAPTED CHILD

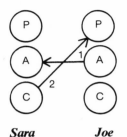

Sara   **Joe**

1. JOE (Adult):
No thanks, I've had enough.

2. SARA (Adapted Child/Persecutor):
I worked all day preparing a nice dinner and now you don't want to eat.

Case

When I met Arlie at an introductory transactional analysis workshop, I was taken immediately by her beauty (auburn hair, twinkling green eyes, and pretty face) which shone through 220 pounds of fat. Pictures taken on her wedding day showed that in 8 years she had transformed from a beauty to a blimp.

Arlie's husband Otto did not care that she was obese; in fact, he seemed to like it. Arlie felt isolated because they seldom went out now but rationalized her social inactivity by babysitter cost.

Her feeling of isolation stimulated Arlie, over Otto's opposition, to reenter the secretarial work force. Getting out into the world caused Arlie to look at her condition. She wanted to change, but each time she tried to lose weight, Otto bought ice cream, pizza, or chocolates to disrupt her diet.

Arlie described Otto as a hard-working man who doted on her and the children. His only serious weakness was excessive jealousy. When they were younger, he had even threatened to strike a man who had stroked Arlie with an appreciative whistle. Otto often talked about his beautiful mother, who had been killed in an automobile owned by a man with whom she was having an affair. Otto felt that his father was destroyed by the knowledge of his wife's unfaithfulness. Otto projected his learned feelings into "women can't be trusted."

Arlie and Otto were playing "Chastity Belt." Arlie said, "Otto seems happy and more secure lately except when I am trying to diet. I feel as if I'm caught in a spider web. The more I struggle to get out, the more securely the web holds on. If I don't do something soon, I'll smother."

Arlie no longer plays "Chastity Belt." She has made an Adult decision to take complete responsibility for her condition.

Otto admits that at first he only agreed to attend a transactional analysis group because he did not want Arlie to go alone. He had mistaken the abbreviation TA for "T Group," or sensitivity training, as portrayed in the Bob and Carol, Ted and Alice movie. He has overcome his initial feelings about transactional analysis and is busy investigating his recordings which say, "Never trust a beautiful woman."

Arlie could have refused to play "Chastity Belt" even if Otto had not joined her study group, but there would have been family disruptions as Otto attempted to keep the belt locked in place. Fortunately, Otto's jealousy caused him to follow her to the group and to learn more about himself and what he was doing to Arlie. Whenever possible, the not-O.K. mate who initiates "Chastity Belt" should be included in the learning program.

Case

Morris reported that he had reduced his excessive eating at mealtimes and had eliminated snacks but had not lost weight. Loretta had reacted forcefully when he cut down his eating, but it was not a major issue now. Instead, she was cooking some tasty new dishes.

Morris recalled that during the previous two weeks he had enjoyed stroganoff, hasenpfeffer, creamed and scalloped vegetables, clam chowder, pecan pie, and a whipped cream sauce on spice cake. A comparison with Morris's previous diet indicated that he had reduced his food intake but not the fat-developing ingredients.

Loretta's new recipes included cream, starch, butter, fat, and sugar, which kept the "Chastity Jock" locked in place. Her Little Professor had developed a strategy that replaced force with manipulation. By switching her recipes, Loretta was getting the same results without the upsetting arguments.

Morris has tried to share his concerns with Loretta. So far she has not accepted transactional analysis as useful and considers it to be a destructive influence.

Morris often asks the group for advice on what to do about Loretta's hang-ups. He is uncomfortable with the answer that Loretta is responsible for how she behaves and feels and that he is responsible for himself. Morris has sufficient problems with fat fever without shouldering Loretta's burden of fear, insecurity, and mistrust. No one can be helped who does not want help. Loretta will change only when she makes an Adult decision that a change is necessary and warranted. Trying to force a change, manipulate involvement, or "shout it out" is a waste of time and effort.

If we accept the premise that a person is responsible for his or her total being, then it is unethical to force change on another individual. Providing Adult information and establishing an environment which supports change is O.K. behavior, but saying "change because I don't like you the way you are" is not only unethical but may very well be impossible. People change when they are ready to change, not when they are directed to change.

"Gray-Coated Savior"

Many obese persons fail in dieting because they have a warped perception of doctors. In the early stages of treatment, the patient perceives the doctor as the Helping Parent/Rescuer. The emotional impact from the treatment influences a change in perception. Perceiving the physician as the Controlling Parent/Persecutor is a usual switch: "I'm afraid to keep my appointment with Dr. O'Connor. He'll raise hell. He told me to lose 10 pounds and I've gained 4 instead. I'd better cancel the appointment."

Recognizing a physician as a Controlling or Helping Parent is normal for most people. Our folklore puts doctors on a level with saviors. One has only to turn on a television medical program to see a white-coated savior correctly diagnosing and treating rare diseases and dispensing valued advice on a variety of subjects.

Most obese persons will follow a physician's instructions for a few days or weeks, but eventually the white coat turns to gray and the patient is back in the old "eat more" pattern. The physician provided Adult professional advice but the patient heard it coming from the Helping or Controlling Parent. While the patient follows the diet, he or she is an Adapted Child/ Victim looking for a Helping Parent/Rescuer who will support the disruption in the diet or reinforce the patient's feeling that the physician's advice is not appropriate. One obese man said, "My doctor is using a gun on me—100 pounds or your life." When he was asked what he was going to do, he replied, "Get another doctor."

Most physicians provide effective Adult advice on the exercise and the diets needed to control the symptoms but cannot provide the hours needed to counsel patients on the psychological basis of fat fever. It is simple to prescribe a cure for the symptoms but difficult to get patients to follow the prescription. Obesity is one of the most frustrating diseases facing physicians as patients refuse to follow the prescription thus very few reach a lasting cure.

Case

Judy has been obese for over 20 years during which time she has played "Gray-Coated Savior" with a number of physicians. When her obesity gets the better of her, Judy visits a physician to cry about this self-inflicted wound. For a few weeks, she follows the physician's advice, but as the white coat turns gray, the Kitchen pattern takes over again. Judy rationalizes her actions by excuses about family and social pressures combined with criticism of the prescribed diet. Any form of confrontation by a physician stimulates Judy to locate another player to be her Gray-Coated Savior.

Finally, Judy located a Rescuer physician who plays by her

rules. He admits her to a hospital yearly, ostensibly for her nerves, during which time she is starved. She leaves the hospital with a prescribed diet which she follows for a few weeks only. As soon as Judy's weight becomes unbearable, her Rescuer admits her back into the hospital. Judy describes her doctor as a wonderful man who really understands her problem. In her game, Judy plays both the Persecutor and the Victim although she blames the Persecutor role on hereditary and physical factors. The doctor is the Helping Parent/Rescuer as he provides a crutch instead of an Adult-designed cure.

It is unusual for a game to last as long as this one (4 years) without a role switch. Judy enjoys her Adapted Child/Victim role and found a physician who enjoys the Helping Parent/ Rescuer role. They deserve each other.

"Midnight Marauder"

A common approach to dealing with obesity is for a significant person (parents, spouse, family member, friend, or some significant other) to force a diet on the overweight person. Sometimes there is no real force exerted, but the patient perceives the significant person as forceful and the results are similar.

Persons enforcing a diet consider that they are operating from the Helping Parent/Rescuer but their actions are perceived by the Adapted Child/Victim as coming from the Controlling Parent/Persecutor.

In some cases, the significant person is trapped into a game by the fat fever sufferer who says: "While I'm on this diet, I'll need your help. If I'm cheating on the diet, I want you to stop me." In other cases, the significant person initiates and forces the game by saying: "I got this new diet from my secretary. It worked for her and I want you to try it. I'll keep the calorie count and ensure that you comply with the diet. I know you don't like diets, but I'm doing this for your own good."

As the game builds in intensity, the Adapted Child/Victim

finds the pressure from the Controlling Parent/Persecutor to be too much to endure passively and thus searches for a Rescuer. When another person cannot be forced to assume the Rescuer role, the Victim switches into the Little Professor to become his or her own Rescuer. The Little Professor develops strategies designed to disrupt the diet.

The Little Professor manipulates the game by sneaking food, nibbling as the roast is being cut, or hiding food and eating it in unusual places such as the garage or bathroom. These Little Professor actions are similar to an alcoholic's behavior when access to liquor is being controlled.

Some Controlling Parent/Persecutors take their role so seriously that it is difficult for the Little Professor to manipulate diet-breaking activities during the day. Close daytime observation forces the Little Professor to play "Midnight Marauder." Refrigerators and cupboards are raided while the Persecutor is asleep.

The Midnight Marauder is difficult to detect. The strategy is to remove small amounts of each food and bypass items which can be counted or noticed easily. Foods in covered packages or boxes (cookies, rainsins, ice cream) or large pieces from which smaller ones can be cut (roast, cheese, salami) are the usual targets. The booty is seldom consumed in the kitchen. It is eaten in the Midnight Marauder's bedroom or in the bathroom if the bedroom is not private enough.

Night snackers usually leave dishes, cutlery, food, and crumbs around, but the Midnight Marauder cleans up very carefully to cover the tracks of the raid. The Marauder puts dishes and cutlery in the dishwasher or washes them, wipes off counters and tables, wraps food carefully, and puts everything back in place.

Although some of the booty is consumed immediately, the Midnight Marauder hides enough food to get through the next day. The hiding places selected are similar to the creative storage areas selected by an alcoholic. Linen closets, drawers, medicine cabinets, tool boxes, clothes closets, car trunks, glove compartments, behind books, top shelves, inside sewing machines, under beds, and under pillows are some of the more usual hiding places.

Case

Claudia was dieting and had asked Hector to stop her if she went off the diet. Because Hector was home recuperating from an illness, he could watch her carefully. There was no evidence that Claudia was breaking her diet, yet she was not losing weight. When Hector confronted her about the "Midnight Marauder" game, Claudia became angry, "How can you doubt me, didn't I ask you to stop me from eating? If I wanted to eat, why would I ask you to help me?" Hector thought he was the Helping Parent/ Rescuer, but Claudia saw him as the Controlling Parent/ Persecutor. Finally Claudia burst into tears: "I try so hard yet you don't trust me. I want to look nice for you. You don't help much. All I get is accusations and hell no matter how hard I try." Claudia was setting up the move to switch Hector to be the Adapted Child/Victim. Instead Hector started a Controlling Parent/Persecutor search for Claudia's food cache.

Claudia took advantage of Hector's unsuccessful search by talking about trust, empathy, suspicion, and other "motherhood" statements. Hector felt bad and sorry for his actions and assumed the Victim role. The more he apologized the more Claudia made him dangle on the barbed Victim hook.

The next day, as Hector set the grandfather clock, he found a bag of gingersnaps and caramels below the weights. He started a second search in more unusual places and found a store of goodies in the snow tires which were stored in the garage. With the new evidence, the roles switched once again and Claudia reverted to the Adapted Child/Victim.

The "Midnight Marauder" game has hidden objectives:

• To show that the fat person cannot lose weight no matter how much he or she diets. The rationale is that it must be a glandular or some other medical problem which the doctor can't identify.

• To prove to the Controlling Parent/Persecutor that the new wonder diet does not work. The fat person is saying, "I told you so."

"Midnight Marauder" players are identifiable by their crooked comments:

• I ate only 900 calories a day for 14 days and did not lose weight.

• Everything I eat is measured but I can't lose weight.

• Shelley controls my diet and she knows I don't cheat.

• I don't eat sweets, fats, or starches. I eat lean meat, salads, and vegetables in small portions but still gain weight.

• I never eat breakfast and often miss lunch. My dinner is only average-sized, yet I can't reduce.

• I've tried every known diet. Maybe I need a gland operation or a stomach bypass.

An individual who forces diets on another person is saying, "I'm O.K.—You're not O.K. You are fat. You need a Rescuer or a Persecutor. I'll help you even if I have to force compliance. You'll thank me someday."

People who assume the Rescuer/Persecutor role enjoy the power it gives them over the overweight individual. The problem with this type of power and authority is that it stimulates dependence which weakens the patient further and reinforces the not-O.K. feeling.

An obese person who initiates the game by asking another person to help or control is saying, "I'm not O.K.—You're O.K. I am pretending I need your help so that you will take an interest in me. The more we play the game, the more you will recognize me. I realize that most of the time I'll be receiving cold or zigzag strokes, but no one strokes me because I'm fat. I'd rather have warm strokes but cold or zigzag strokes are better than none."

Almost every obese person who is an on-again–off-again dieter is a Midnight Marauder. The Adult response to an invitation to play "Midnight Marauder" is, "Sorry, no other person can help you diet or lose weight. If you really want to lose weight, you can do it alone." The overweight "Midnight

Marauder" player can suspend the game by an Adult realization that people who really want to lose weight refuse to play games.

"Maternity"

Some women wear very loose clothing or maternity-type outfits to camouflage fat. Young married women who reduce for the mating dance and gain their weight back soon after marriage are often initiators of the "Maternity" game. Friends and relatives are too polite to ask about the condition but observe the maternity clothes and bulges as a sign that a baby is on the way.

"Maternity"-game players rely on vagueness or misleading replies to the question, "When are you due?" "Not for some time yet," or "I'm not sure yet," provides more time and scope to play out the game.

Eventually a "Maternity" player must put up or be unmasked as a phony. It is very unusual for a "Maternity" player to admit that she is not pregnant; thus she acts out elaborate and sometimes costly schemes:

• Resigning a job on the pretext that it is too difficult for her in her condition.

• Transferring within an organization or taking a job elsewhere.

• Going on a starvation diet combined with faking a miscarriage. (One "Maternity" player starved herself during her vacation and reported a miscarriage. Her co-workers were sympathetic: "Poor Georgia, she is trying so hard to have a baby and can't hold it. That was her third miscarriage.")

• Deciding a real pregnancy is the only way out, even though she has no desire for a baby, and setting up the game strategy by neglecting birth control.

• Isolating herself from co-workers, friends, and relatives in order to delay facing up.

Women who play "Maternity" have a history of significant others' persecuting them about weight. When a young woman from a weight-conscious family gains weight, she knows what the persecuting reaction will be. Her choice is between isolation or deception. Deception, in the form of the "Maternity" game, is the least uncomfortable tactic and may even be a bonus as the player gets warm strokes of compassion, understanding, and thankfulness for being pregnant. Although it feels good to receive the recognition of productivity stroke—"You are a real woman"—strokes based on deception are disruptive to internal peace.

The obese Victim knows from experience that people persecute for fatness. Her Kitchen pattern programs her to eat until she panics. The appropriate move would be an Adult plan based on logic, fact, and reason, but instead her emotional fear pushes her into the manipulative, deceptive Little Professor. The Little Professor says, "You need time; hide your weight by loose clothing." Loose clothing and a few bulges on a young married woman spell out pregnancy to observers. Although the Victim may not have started out with the "Maternity" game in mind, the Little Professor, grabbing at straws, does nothing to correct the misinterpretation.

"Maternity" is an unusual game in that the roles are suppressed. The obese woman perceives other people as Persecutors even though they are inactive. She believes that they would persecute if they realized that fat, not pregnancy, was hidden beneath the maternity dress. The Helping Parent/Rescuer does not come forward because no need for a Rescuer is indicated; after all, pregnancy is O.K. The obese woman feels more and more victimized as the game progresses and uses even more manipulation to extricate herself. On occasion the husband becomes a Rescuer willingly or unwillingly through a real pregnancy. When this happens, the husband may feel like a Victim, especially if their marriage plans are based on two incomes, not a lone provider.

Case

Valerie had lost 40 pounds prior to her mating dance. After 6 months of married life, she started to gain weight and shifted to loose-fitting clothing as a deception. She responded with vagueness, curtness, and flippancy to comments about pregnancy, but nevertheless after 2 months she was wearing maternity clothes and accepting the little kindnesses accorded the pregnant woman.

Bob and Valerie had planned to delay starting a family for 3 years so that they could save enough for a down payment on a house. Bob was surprised when Valerie told him that she was pregnant and that she would have to stop working in a few months. Unknown to Bob, Valerie had stopped taking the pill with the objective of rescuing herself by a real pregnancy. Bob felt victimized by fate now that their plans were disrupted.

Two weeks later Valerie told Bob that she had to stop working immediately because of back pains and other complications. She had contrived the pains so that she could get away from her co-workers who thought she was 6 months pregnant rather than 2½ months. Bob felt even more victimized now that her salary would stop almost immediately rather than in 5 or 6 months. His Victim feeling was reinforced further when living expenses and the car payment necessitated his moonlighting at a gas station.

Valerie is now 7 months pregnant and looks like a hippopotamus. As she sits and shovels chocolates into her face, she blames her size on pregnancy. Women who play "Maternity" and finally are rescued by a real pregnancy are deceiving themselves when they think childbirth will reduce obesity. The outcome is more likely to be a continuing and increased case of fat fever.

"Maternity" players attempt to manipulate their husbands into accepting responsibility for the wife's obesity.

• I was never fat before I had the baby.
• Something happened in childbirth which stops me from losing weight.
• I had a lovely shape before. Just look at what you did to me.

The strategy is to make the husband assume responsibility so that any move on his part to bail out will be counteracted by guilt. Many husbands who would like to get away from an obese wife do not leave because they feel guilty.

"Fat Mother"

Fat women often trade their "sorry" stamps in ways similar to the "torn-mother" syndrome. The torn mother makes a child feel guilty by exaggerating the horrors of childbirth. "Why, when you were born, you were so big and I was so small that I had 400 stitches and had to stay in bed for 12 weeks. You tore me open." In the "Fat Mother" game she says, "I was 118 pounds before you were born. Pregnancy disrupted the balance of my glands so that I'll always be fat. Here, look at me in a bathing suit the year before you were born." Many people carry guilt rackets throughout their lives due to parents' using the "torn-mother" syndrome or "Fat Mother" game.

Rarely is childbirth responsible for continuing obesity. Although I have heard women laying on guilt via the "Fat Mother" game, I have not yet seen much evidence to support their contention. One interesting observation is that out of six women who admitted using the "Fat Mother" game on their children, five recalled their own mother using the torn-mother syndrome on them.

The Parent ego state learns and adapts strategies for destructive transference of guilt and other rackets to the unsuspecting and receptive children who end up living with a racket which is not based on reality or fact.

"Blame"

There are other fat fever games which can be classified by their blame of someone else. The obese Victim perceives another person as the Persecutor who provides or stimulates excessive consumption of food and drink. The objective of "Blame" is to switch the roles so that the obese person can make excuses for being fat and transfer the blame to another person. The fat blamer switches to a Persecutor role to make the other person feel like a guilty Victim.

"Blame" games are usually of short duration with a number of rapid switches. The obese person tries to assume a power position by blaming, and the blamee attempts to ward off the thrusts by rationalization, hostility, or changing the game.

"See What You Made Me Do"

"See What You Made Me Do" players are saying, "I didn't want to eat but you made me do it. You are to blame for my condition. If I were isolated from you I could lose weight."

Financially able Victims who feel that they require isolation to reduce are prime candidates for health spas and residential weight-control clinics. Stringent diet and exercise at the clinic take off weight and reinforce the Victim's feelings that the at-home Persecutor is responsible for his or her obesity. In reality, the Victim has only switched Persecutors, as the clinic, by one means or another, is the Controlling Parent forcing weight loss. By paying for the treatment, the customer is likely to feel comfortable about the clinic experience, perceiving it as a Helping Parent/Rescuer activity.

The fat fever patient then returns home and says, "I told you so. I was away from you for 3 weeks and lost 14 pounds." Unfortunately, once away from the Controlling Parent clinic, the Victim gains back the lost weight and "See What You Made Me Do" is reinitiated. Eventually the Victim returns to the Controlling Parent clinic for another period of isolation. The clinic may have an effective program but has no way to ensure that the patient continues the treatment at home. Some clinic operators are pleased that the cure does not last, for the basis of their business is customers' returning for more isolation.

Players who cannot pay for isolation may continue the game until it gets too repressive. The isolation payoff comes when the other player finds every excuse imaginable to come home late or stay away as much as possible.

Some players have a Gray-Coated Savior who provides the isolation payoff by admitting them to a hospital. This is similar to the use of weight-control clinics except that the financial burden is borne by health insurance and the state.

"If It Weren't For You"

"If It Weren't For You" players react from the Adapted Child Victim role but do not see another person's using force as in "See What You Made Me Do." "If It Weren't For You" players blame their condition on the habits, behavior, and weaknesses of other people.

- If it weren't for your eating a bedtime snack, I wouldn't eat one.
- If it weren't for your loving pizza, I wouldn't have it so often.
- If it weren't for your sweet tooth, I would never buy ice cream or candy.
- If it weren't for your gifts of chocolates, I would never eat them.
- If it weren't for your eating three large meals a day, I wouldn't eat very much.
- If it weren't for your making me feel bad, I wouldn't eat extra.
- If it weren't for your missing dinner so often, I wouldn't finish the leftovers.

The player is saying, "I am a fat fever Victim because as I react to meet your needs, I persecute myself by eating excessively. You can Rescue me by changing your behavior and habits so that I will not be stimulated to eat."

"I Am Only Trying To Help You"

"I Am Only Trying To Help You" is a game which is initiated from a Helping Parent/Rescuer role.

FRANK (Little Professor/Hungry Victim): My throat is a bit sore, I wonder what would relieve the dryness.

JOY (Helping Parent/Rescuer): Your voice does sound harsh. A dish of maple walnut ice cream may relieve you a bit.

FRANK (Controlling Parent/Persecutor): Damn it, you're stupid. You know I am dieting. Why did you have to give me ice cream? I'll never lose weight around here.

JOY (Adapted Child/Victim): I didn't mean to break your diet but your throat was sore. I am only trying to help you.

FRANK (Controlling Parent/Persecutor): "Some help. You are destroying me. You know I have a promotion board in three weeks and I want to look good. Why don't you think once in a while?

JOY (Adapted Child/Victim): I'm sorry. Every time I try to help you, I get abuse. I'm going to bed.

Frank's Little Professor hooked Joy's Helping Parent. After enjoying the ice cream, Frank started the switch by playing "See What You Made Me Do." Frank was setting up a future move in the "Blame" game by referring to the promotion board. If he doesn't get the promotion, he will be able to attribute his lack of success on weight and victimize Joy again. The game may go on for some time, as Frank continues to shirk his responsibility by making Joy feel guilty over and over again.

"Get The World Off My Shoulders"

"Get The World Off My Shoulders" is a fat fever game initiated by a Victim who feels the weight of the world's problems. The day-to-day issues become too much to bear, so the fat fever Victim uses excessive food and drink for self-persecution. The Victim feels that the self-destructive course can be changed only if a Rescuer appears who can solve and/or remove the pressures.

"Get The World Off My Shoulders" players use each and every incident no matter how minor, as an excuse to eat: The kids were bad today; Harry was grumpy; Mother talked too much; I worked so hard; the neighbor's dog barked all day; Jill stayed out past ten o'clock; Peter failed algebra; Father yelled at me; the power went off in the middle of my soap opera; Mary didn't invite me to her tea; the cat dug up my petunias.

"I'm Doing This For Your Own Good"

"I'm Doing This For Your Own Good" is initiated by a Controlling Parent/Persecutor who tells the Adapted Child/Victim how much or how little to eat. The Persecutor sees the Victim as Not O.K. and says, "I have to save you from yourself." In most cases the game initiator considers himself or herself to be a Helping Parent/Rescuer, but the Victim perceives the behavior as Controlling Parent/Persecutor.

The hostility, anger, bad feelings, and hurt associated with "I'm Doing This For Your Own Good" are accentuated by the different perceptions of the role. Mother forcing children to eat up sees it as the action of the Helping Parent, but the children see it as the Controlling Parent. When a husband sets a diet for his wife, he sees himself as helping, but the wife perceives it as power, control, and authority. When the Victim reacts aggressively, the initiator can't understand because "After all, I'm doing this for your own good; you'll thank me someday." The Victim who is being forced to eat or forced to diet may comply for short periods but will develop tactics and strategies to disrupt the game at the expense of the initiator, who ends up the not-O.K. Victim.

The "I'm Doing This For Your Own Good" player seldom gets the someday thanks. The fat fever Victim cannot be forced to diet. Diets come from internal needs, not external force. On the other hand, "I'm Doing This For Your Own Good" players who force food on children are usually coming from a Kitchen pattern and may successfully Kitchen-program the child. The child cannot fight the big person, and therefore accepts an adaptation which becomes part of a destructive program.

"Easter Egg"

Some Helping Parent/Rescuers hide special-treat foods from

the Victim dieter, much as whiskey is hidden from an alcoholic or cigarets from a person trying to stop smoking. The reasoning is that when special-treat foods are out of reach, the Victim is being helped and protected. As the dieter carries on normal activities, he or she may find the Easter Egg cache by chance and, as everyone knows, when a child finds an Easter Egg, it is his or hers to eat.

If the Victim is aware that special-treat foods are hidden away, the Easter Egg hunt is on as soon as the diet becomes too much to bear. Once found, some of the food cache will be eaten up and the remainder moved to a safer hiding place for a rainy day.

It is interesting to see fat fever Victims hide special-treat foods away and pretend to forget where they are stored. Victims then rescue themselves by stumbling onto the cache or by having a pretend Easter Egg hunt. It may be more descriptive for this variation of "Easter Egg" to be called "Pack Rat."

"Celebration"

"Celebration" is a fat fever game initiated by the Little Professor. The dieting Victim searches for reasons to celebrate a special event. The celebration becomes the rescuing activity as, after all, no one is expected to diet on special occasions.

It is reasonable to celebrate birthdays, wedding anniversaries, graduations, promotions, and other important events, but the "Celebration" players go too far. The range of events selected for the "Celebration" game are creative and sometimes amusing:

 • A pet's (dog, cat, bird) birthday.
 • Friendship or one of the other specified national weeks.
 • Parents' anniversaries and birthdays even after they are deceased.
 • Sammy's passing his arithmetic test.
 • Anniversay of a "first" of something—the day we met, our first date, etc.

• Children's birthdays even when they are miles away and can't attend.

• One fat fever sufferer celebrates the anniversary of her three marriages as well as the anniversary of her two divorces.

"Jolly Fat Fred"

"Jolly Fat Fred" (or Freda) is an adaptation from the Parent tapes which tells the obese person that fat people are jolly, humorous, pleasant people meant to be jokers and entertainers. Nursery rhymes, fairy tales, children's stories, comics, movies, and television show the fat man as happy and smiling. Fiction often portrays the fat man as a winner compared to the morose, stoic thin-man loser. The image of the winner fat man is reinforced by television programs such as "Cannon" (a fat private-eye hero) and the "Dumplings" comic strip which describes a winner marriage between two fat people.

Playing out the roles in "Jolly Fat Fred" is a destructive influence on fat fever sufferers. As they pretend to enjoy fatness, obese people are manipulating themselves to live with their disease instead of curing it. Fat people assume the Controlling Parent/Persecutor role by applying fat-humor to themselves, the Adapted Child/Victim.

Both the fat man and the recipient of the humor may consider themselves to be in the Free Child, but it is not realistic to accept destructive behavior as the natural, fun-loving Child. The recipient is a combination of Controlling Parent/Persecutor—"As I laugh at you, you will keep up the game and eventually destroy yourself"—and the Helping Parent/Rescuer—"As I laugh with you, you'll feel better." No matter how hard and how often the game players laugh, the people playing along with "Jolly Fat Fred" are coming mostly from the Persecutor role because of the gallows transactions and the continuing negative fat fever payoffs from the game.

The switch in "Jolly Fat Fred" comes when some other person gets caught up in the game and makes remarks or tells jokes reflecting on the fat person or on weight. Fat people see this as persecuting behavior and react by anger, sarcasm, rudeness, and even assault. The perceived antagonist becomes the unhappy Victim. The number of times that this switch occurs suggests that the "Jolly Fat Fred" uses the game to trade in resentment stamps.

One "Jolly Fat Fred" player reacted to questions about his moves with, "My grandfather was fat and jolly. My father was fat and jolly. So I have to be fat and jolly." His Parent message was, "Be fat and jolly like us," and his Adapted Child accepted the message and played out the game plan. He had to make an Adult decision that removed the "I have to be" message. One colleague helped when he said, "Your grandfather died at 43 and your father at 45, both from heart attacks. Does that mean you have only 8 to 10 years to go?" The realization that he was playing out a death role and could make an Adult-based change influenced our "Jolly Fat Fred" to make the change to the "Happy Winner."

"Nellie The Nibbler"

Many fat fever sufferers play "Nellie (or Nelson) The Nibbler" from what they believe to be a Helping Parent/ Rescuer. "I'm a little hungry—a few peanuts, potato chips, or whatever, won't hurt me." "I'm not really nibbling—just tasting the dinner to see if it's done yet; all cooks have to taste first." The rationale is that nibbles don't count.

"Nellie The Nibbler" may not eat excessively at mealtimes and may even give the appearance of maintaining a diet. The Nibbler is both the Persecutor and the Victim in the game. The excessive food intake attributable to nibbling is reducing the Victim's chance for a healthy life. The Victim looks around for a Rescuer from the diet or other restraints. "Look at me, Charlie. I eat less than you do, yet I'm gaining weight." She would like Rescuer Charlie to say, "Nuts to dieting, Nellie. When you're unhappy, I'm unhappy. Knock it off." Most people who are rescued in this way continue to gain weight until they go into depression about how they feel and look. A usual play is to blame Charlie: "Why did you make me stop dieting? I look so ugly, I could kill myself." Rescuer Charlie ends up the Victim and Nellie becomes the Persecutor again as well as continuing as the fat fever Victim.

Some nibblers want to be and expect to be caught. They nibble along knowing full well that Persecutor Charlie will say, "Hell, you don't eat much. You nibble all day long. No wonder your diet doesn't work. You'd better get with the diet or you won't see much of me." The resulting uproar provides Nellie with a new reason for eating more, and Charlie can be blamed for upsetting her so that she had to eat.

Nibblers hang around the kitchen while food is being prepared to taste the roast, lick the frosting spoon, try an oatmeal cookie, or pick at the salad bowl. One evening a young visitor, an on-again–off-again dieter, was in our kitchen as my wife prepared dinner. She tried each course as she talked to Joy and nibbled what I calculated to be about 800 calories. At dinner, she refused strawberry shortcake because of her very strict diet, even though she had eaten several strawberries and cleaned the whipped-cream bowl before dinner. She was acting out "See What a Good Girl Am I" and was rewarded by a stroke from her husband who had not seen "Nellie The Nibbler" in action.

Obese people usually play Nellie The Nibbler while they are preparing food. When a woman says, "I never eat much when I prepare meals but really enjoy a meal when I'm out," there is a 99 percent chance that she plays "Nellie The Nibbler" while she is in her own kitchen.

Another "Nellie The Nibbler" strategy is to prepare a snack for a nondieting visitor or family member and then sit back in the "See What A Good Girl Am I" or "Martyr" pose as the nondieter eats up. Nellie is able to sit and watch because she nibbled her fill as she prepared the snack. But of course, nibbles don't count, especially if you eat fast and don't get caught.

"Put Off"

"Put Off" is a "Yes, But" game played by obese people who do not really want to lose weight. They ask for help but react to each recommendation or suggestion with a plausible-appearing No Surprise transaction which carries the hidden message, "I don't want and won't accept your advice. Leave me alone. I'm happy fat, so why upset me?" The payoff is isolation and continued obesity.

MERV (Helpless Child/Victim): I sure would like to reduce. You were successful. Can you help me?

RAY (Helping Parent/Rescuer): I used transactional analysis. A 3-day workshop will help you.

MERV (Adult-sounding helpless Child/Victim): I would like to try TA, but I can't afford the 3 days or the cost of a workshop.

RAY (Helping Parent/Rescuer): I'll lend you *Born To Win;* it's easy to read. Maybe that will give you a start until you can afford a workshop.

MERV (Helpless Child/Victim): I don't think that would be much good. I tried reading a TA book and didn't think much of it. Maybe TA is too deep for me.

RAY (Helping Parent/Rescuer): Possibly you could read a chapter at a time and we could discuss it to ensure that you are getting the correct message.

MERV (Adult-sounding helpless Child/Victim): Yes, that's a possibility, but I can't spare the time now.

Merv was telling Ray, "I've asked for your help but there isn't anything you can suggest or recommend that I will accept." If Ray's internal messages say, "Be a helper and a Rescuer," or, "Saviors and missionaries don't give up," he will continue to play "Put Off" by providing additional advice, recommendations, and suggestions. Otherwise, he will withdraw from the game as soon as his Adult reasons, "Everything I say gets a 'Yes, But.' The 'Put Off' game is too frustrating. Merv doesn't want help, so why bother?"

When Ray withdraws from the game by withholding his help, Merv will be able to say, "I'm on my own. No one cares enough to help me. I'll die fat." Merv remains in a helpless, resentful position until he identifies a new Rescuer who is interested in playing "Put Off."

"Worry Wart"

The "Worry Wart" game is initiated by a significant other person who tries to operate from a Helping Parent/Rescuer. The objective is to make the obese person feel guilty about the worry being caused and to react as an Adapted Child/Victim. The Rescuer is saying, "When you lose weight, I'll be able to feel O.K. again. If you continue on as you are, the worry will kill me."

Most obese people are not willing to adapt to the Rescuer's plea and may even react with anger and hostility. This allows the Rescuer to switch to the Controlling Parent/Persecutor who attempts to force and control eating and weight-related activities. The Victim then searches for a Rescuer who will get the Persecutor off the Victim's back.

The "Worry Wart" game is played often by a mother who is worried and embarrassed that her fat daughter will be an old maid. The game is played until the father finally takes on the Rescuer role to protect the daughter from the controlling mother. Many fathers assume the Rescuer role willingly from an internal drive to keep their daughters at home and single. This is a form of "Chastity Belt" for the father who feels that fat daughters are less trouble and are more likely to stay home to comfort dear old Dad.

The game continues with a role switch. Father persecutes Mother, the new Victim, for her insensitive behavior about weight, and the fight is on. Daughter watches "Let's You and Him Fight" until the uproar gets too serious; then she rejoins the game to rescue poor Mother, who was only trying to help.

The "Worry Wart" game is identified by the initiator's statements:

- I worry because I love you.

- I worry that you will be an old maid.
- I worry that you are so fat.
- I worry that you eat so much.
- I worry that you do not have a date for the dance.
- I worry what will happen to you when I'm gone.
- I worry that you don't have the willpower to diet.

The worrier who says, "My only worry is Sally's weight," is fooling himself or herself. If there is no fat daughter, Worry Warts will find something else to worry about. Worriers enjoy reexperiencing the worry feelings, which is an adaptation from early life. The Worry Wart feels "I'm O.K.—You're not O.K.," but continuous playing of the "Worry Wart" game and/or racket means that the player really feels, "Underneath my cosmetics I'm not O.K. either." O.K. people do not get hooked into protracted periods of worrying because their Adults tell them that worrying is a nonproductive, personally destructive feeling.

The "Worry Wart" game is unsuccessful in programming a permanent weight reduction. The change comes only when the obese person makes an Adult decision to change. Inevitably, Rescuer worriers become Victims because fear, guilt, and other "rackety" feelings are the internal tools of losers, not winners.

"NIGYSOB"

"NIGYSOB" (Now I've got you, you S.O.B.) players enjoy fat fever games. The NIGYSOBer pretends to help and rescue the obese target by setting limits, rules, procedures, and guidelines on diets, exercise, and other food-related issues. The NIGYSOBer really enjoys the Controlling Parent/Persecutor role. He or she sets impractical food-control limits, then tempts the Victim to break the limits by making desirable food easily available or by discussing food and recipes and by snacking in front of the drooling Victim.

The NIGYSOBer watches the Victim carefully and may even allow minor transgressions. Eventually, the Victim makes a major infraction and the Persecutor comes down hard with both feet, using anger, criticism, and even physical punishment, which increases the Victim's feelings of guilt, fear, and depression. The NIGYSOBer set up the game so that he or she could enjoy the power and authority of "Now I've got you, you S.O.B."

"Kick Me"

"Kick Me," a game similar to NIGYSOB, is initiated by an obese person who asks for help and direction from a Controlling Parent. The parties agree on the limits, Kitchen rules, and enforcement obligations. The Victim then sets up the game by breaking the rules and leaving enough evidence for apprehension by the Controlling Parent/Persecutor.

The Victim sets up situations which attract emotional and physical punishment. He or she is saying, "I want to be caught. I want you to punish me. I get my strokes by being kicked. When you kick me, I know you care or at least know that I am here."

The theoretical differences between "NIGYSOB" and "Kick Me" are:

• The Persecutor initiates "NIGYSOB," sets up the traps, and enjoys kicking.

• The Victim initiates "Kick Me," leaves evidence to ensure apprehension, and enjoys being kicked.

The two games are so similar in moves and impact that "NIGYSOB" is often mistaken for "Kick Me" and vice-versa. I support the TA differentiations because it is important to identify from which hand a game is played and the major motivations of the players.

ELIMINATING FAT FEVER GAMES

It is not practical and it may be even impossible to eliminate all psychological games from our lives.

• Stroke-deprived people get recognition by playing games.
• Bored people pass time by playing games.
• Not-O.K. people reinforce their life positions and family

patterns and reexperience their "rackety" feelings through games.

• It is a very rare person who is so O.K. that he or she has no need for games. Everyone plays games of one type or another, but O.K. people play fewer, less intense, less destructive games.

A permanent fat fever cure is possible only if destructive fat fever games are eliminated. One should not expect to cancel out all the games immediately. Games are as much a part of an individual as a big toe. It may be more realistic to eliminate the most destructive games first and to decrease, disrupt, and postpone other games until we can cope with the psychological reactions to such a major change.

It is simple to plan to eliminate games, but it is difficult to do, especially when they are part of a Kitchen pattern. Our physical and psychological being is weaned on games. We learn our games, our roles, the strategies, the tactics, and the moves. The requirements for game elimination are:

• Familiarity with games and game theory.

• Practice in game identification.

• Awareness of one's own favorite games, rackets, ego states, and roles.

• Identification of one's own primary and secondary family pattern.

• Ability to recognize and ward off the barbed Parent and Child hooks and the ulterior messages which invite players into the game.

• Ability to stay in the Adult and to say, "No, I won't play, no matter how tempting the invitation may be."

• Action to eliminate Drama roles of Rescuer, Persecutor, and Victim.

• Learning to live without getting or giving the negative payoffs which are the outcome of games.

• Action to reduce stamp collections and destructive trading.

• Emphasis on warm strokes and elimination of cold and zigzag strokes.

EXERCISE: GAMES I PLAY

1. Circle the names of the fat fever games which you have seen in operation.

"Chastity Belt"
"Gray-Coated Savior"
"Maternity"
"Midnight Marauder"
"See What You Made Me Do"
"If It Weren't For You"
"Easter Egg"
"Celebration"
"Kick Me"

"I Was Only Trying To Help You"
"Get The World Off My Shoulders"
"I'm Doing This For Your Own Good"
"Jolly Fat Fred"
"Nellie The Nibbler"
"Put Off"
"Worry Wart"
"NIGYSOB"

2. Decide on a descriptive, "catchy" name for other fat fever games which you have observed.

3. Select and describe the moves in one fat fever game which is played at your home, your work, or among your friends. From which ego state and drama role is the game initiated? What role do you and others play, including switches? What feelings are collected by the participants, and who gets the negative payoff?

Name of game:_____
Description of game and switching strategy:

Initiator's role: Ego state _____ Drama role _____
Roles you play: (1) Ego state _____ (2) Ego state _____
Drama role _____ Drama role _____
Roles others play: (1) Ego state _____ (2) Ego state _____
Drama role _____ Drama role _____
(3) Ego state _____
Drama role _____
Feelings
collected: (1) _____ (2) _____
(3) _____
Negative payoff: Who _____ What_____

4. The above game recall will indicate how you are structuring your activities to reexperience favored feelings.

What is your favorite game? _____

What is your favorite Drama role? _____

What is your favorite feeling (racket)? _____

How do you show or emphasize your weakness concerning food and weight? _____

How do you show or emphasize the weakness or strength of the most significant other person in your games? _____

5. How do you perceive that the most significant other person in your games would answer these questions? This person should be someone who is with you often, such as husband, wife, father, or mother.

What is his or her favorite game? _____

What is his or her favorite Drama role? _____

What is his or her favorite feeling (racket)? _____

How does he or she emphasize your weakness concerning food and weight? _____

How does he or she emphasize his or her own weakness or strength? _____

6. What corrective action can you take to give up games? Be specific; say what you will do and how you will do it.

7. Based on the recall stimulated by the exercises and your knowledge of your games, please return to Chapter 3 and amend your pattern pizza as required.

CHAPTER

8
Fat Fever Time

Generally, people structure time to meet physical and emotional wants and needs. If we enjoy physical exercises, we may play tennis, jog, or ride a bicycle. If we enjoy passivity and quietness, we may spend hours alone reading and listening to music. Transactional analysts say that we meet these personal desires through:

- Withdrawal
- Pastimes
- Rituals
- Games
- Activities
- Intimacy [1]

Obese individuals use food, drink, diets, and other weight-related issues to structure their use of time. Fat fever sufferers are either eating to excess or on a starvation diet. When their emotional or physical needs become dominant, fat fever sufferers shift to a more acceptable (to them) use of time.

The relationship to time and the structuring of time is programmed in the family pattern.

- When a child says, "There's nothing to do around here," the Kitchen mother says, "Have a piece of bread and brown sugar." The messages received are "Eat when you're bored," and "Food is good for emotional upsets."
- When a child says, "There's nothing to do around here," the Bathroom mother says, "Go and sit on the pottie—you haven't had a good 'do-do' for days." The message received is "Pottie perching cures bad feelings."
- When a child says, "There's nothing to do around here," the Hurt mother says, "Quit bothering me or you'll get a whack

on the behind. Go out and play in the traffic." The message received is "Hostility, violence, and danger cure bad feelings."

• When a child says, "There's nothing to do around here," the Love mother says, "Let's sit down and think of some 'cool' things to do together." The message received is "It's O.K. to be bored, but warmth and understanding will erase bad feelings."

WITHDRAWAL

Withdrawal can be psychological or physical and for long or short periods of time. A hermit physically withdraws for long periods while a father who escapes to his study is withdrawing for a short period. When we daydream, fantasize, or turn off, we are withdrawing psychologically.

Kitchen people use withdrawal as a "living with obesity" tool. Obese people who stay home, refuse social invitations, by-pass social opportunities, isolate themselves from friends and colleagues, avoid getting a picture taken, and are often alone with spouses and children are withdrawing to hide away from the critical glances.

Obese people who fantasize about changing from Dumpy Dora to Curvy Carla or daydream about the transformation from Rolly Raymond to Muscles Marvin are using psychological withdrawal to meet their needs.

Withdrawal is an O.K. behavior when the objective is thinking and relaxation. Withdrawal for reasons of getting away from other people and hiding weight rather than taking Adult action and responsibility is destructive.

The obese person combines excessive eating with withdrawal. The Kitchen pattern says, "Eating will cure boredom, so hide away and eat." The more an obese person withdraws, the less chance there is for a cure.

Exercise: How I Withdraw

1. Describe two incidents when your self-consciousness

about weight influenced you to act in one of the following manners:

• Refuse a chance to celebrate, dance, or socialize.
• Run and hide from the all-seeing camera or cry, "You don't want my picture, I'll break the camera."
• Isolate yourself from people.
• Fantasize and daydream about being slim.

A.

B.

2. Describe one fantasy or daydream in which you saw yourself as slender and beautiful or muscular and athletic. What are you doing and what is the reaction of other people in your fantasy?

3. What is your favorite way of withdrawing?

4. What ego state are you in when you withdraw? Why?

RITUALS

Rituals are No Surprise, recurring transactions, such as:
• Starting a meeting with the club song.

- Ending a meeting with a pledge or lodge oath.
- Passing through a reception line at a wedding or cocktail party.
- Convocation ceremonies, wedding celebrations, and birthday parties.
- Standard activities around which churches, political parties, or social groups structure their time.

Most people recognize the above as rituals but are less likely to see day-to-day social interactions as ritualistic. For example, when Jack says, "Hi, Charlie, what's new?" he expects a ritualistic, "Nothing much, what's new with you?" and not a 30-minute description of a new home. Some other rituals established for social interaction are coffee at ten and three o'clock, brunch on Sunday, and happy hour on Friday.

Programmed rituals stimulate fat fever; some of these are:
- Always having a second serving.
- Eating three meals a day, a ritual originating from the time when most people worked at physical labor.
- Lunch-bagging it Monday to Thursday and eating out on Friday.
- Forcing children to eat.
- The "Celebration" game.
- Drinking cocktails or beer before dinner.
- Having bedtime snacks, doughnuts at coffee breaks, or beer and popcorn while watching television.

The sit-down family dinner is a disappearing ritual. Many people eat junk food on the run and have a sit-down dinner only occasionally. This practice induces fat fever, as junk foods are more fattening than the balanced diet which is more likely at a sit-down dinner.

The pace of contemporary living is disrupting the family dinner ritual. In the modern family, one or more members usually miss meals. Johnny eats a sandwich early because he has a little league ball game. Sally has a snack because she is going to a rock and roll concert. Mother hasn't got the time to cook properly because she has to get ready for a bridge date. Father rushes through dinner because this is his bowling night. It is not possible for family members to eat all their meals together, but the once-a-day family dinner is an important event which should not be ignored.

The family dinner is important for two reasons:

• There is a much greater nutritional value in eating properly rather than snacking. Nutritionists say it is not only how much a person eats but what that person eats which causes obesity.

• Meals are the one time when the whole family is together and mealtime is an important input to a realistic program. As one lady said, "It is difficult to get time to talk to the children now. We seldom eat together any more except when there is a family celebration. I remember working alongside the children when we washed the dinner dishes. There was a lot of bickering, but there was also a lot of talking, listening, and understanding. The automatic dishwasher may save time, but it closes up one important communication opportunity. Eating as a family and washing the dishes together are two rituals which I would like reinstitute in my home."

EXERCISE: RITUALS IN MY LIFE

1. List three rituals which take place in your home, at work, or with friends. Explain how these rituals were initiated and how they influenced fat fever.

A.

B.

C.

2. How can you eliminate or decrease the fat fever effects of your rituals?

GAMES AND RACKETS

People play games and rackets to structure time. "See What You Made Me Do" or "Celebration" may be a short-duration game of a few moments, a few hours, or a few days. Time may be structured around "Maternity" for several months while "Nellie The Nibbler" or "Jolly Fat Fred" may be lifelong fat fever games.

Some potentially fat people start by structuring their time with short-term games, but as fat fever takes hold they adopt more intense, longer duration games.

Exercise: My Games and Time Usage

1. On the basis of your responses to the Chapter 7 *Games I Play* exercise, how do you use games to structure time?

2. Review the development of your game pattern. Did your fat fever games start out as low-intensity, short-duration games? Have you progressed to longer-duration games?

3. What Adult action can you take to restructure your time so that fat fever games are reduced or eliminated?

PASTIMES

Pastimes are the harmless conversations and activities which people use to pass time. Pastimes are exchanges which can be carried out without real involvement and commitment from the participants. Pastime subjects are sports, children, politics, poor service, food prices, hobbies, animals, recreational activities, or any other subject which is safe and does not require in-depth reactions from the involved persons.

Fat fever sufferers integrate their harmless pastimes with harmful overindulgence in food and drink.

• Women passing time discussing the cute sayings of their children may be drinking coffee and eating cupcakes.

• Men discussing sports may be drinking beer and eating buttered popcorn and pretzels.

• Shoppers complaining about food prices may be loading their baskets with potato chips, soda pop, and other junk food.

• People discussing politics may be drinking scotch and eating rich canapés.

• Men discussing their latest golf tournament may be sipping gin and eating peanuts.

EXERCISE: REVIEWING MY PASTIMES

1. On the following chart, list your three favorite pastimes. With whom and when (under what conditions) does the pastime occur? How is each pastime related to fat fever?

Favorite Pastime	With Whom	When/Conditions	Relationship to Fat Fever
1			
2			
3			

2. Is there a pattern to your pastimes? Are your favorite pastimes similar? Are the same people involved? Are the feelings, conditions, time, etc., similar? Is food or drink involved? Are the pastimes passive, nonphysical activities?

3. What can you do to eliminate or reduce the relationship between fat fever stimulators and your pastimes?

ACTIVITIES

Activities are the useful projects or tasks which are productive for ourselves or others, such as:

- Taking piano lessons.
- Participating in a TA group.
- Cutting the grass.
- Attending college.
- Delivering the mail.
- Keeping records.
- Doing housework.
- Selling a product.
- Designing an ad layout.
- Working.

Generally, fat fever sufferers do not have enough productive activities around which to structure their time. The resulting free time is filled by fat-fever-inducing withdrawal, pastimes, rituals, games, and rackets.

People who have a full work life and an active leisure life are usually not serious fat fever victims. An individual who structures time around productive work and self-fulfilling leisure activities and hobbies is less likely to fall into the obesity trap.

Obese people who work around food or who have food-related hobbies often integrate games with their productive activities.

- Jessie plays "Nellie The Nibbler" while she cooks dinner.
- Saul plays "Put Off" when his excuse for obesity is "Yes,

but no one working in a pizza parlor can lose weight."

· Joanie uses her gourmet cooking hobby as an excuse to play "Celebration."

Some people do not have an obesity problem, or at least seem to be in reasonable control of their weight, while they are leading an active life. When activity patterns are disrupted by retirement, illness, unemployment, changes in social or family life, or changes in employment, some people restructure their time around games, rackets, pastimes, rituals, and withdrawal, which stimulates fat fever.

Case

Once the children were off to school, Lorrie had time on her hands. Afternoon tea and sweets with the girls progressed to bridge and the "My Dessert Is Better Than Yours" game. The desire to fill up free time made Lorrie a fat fever victim.

Case

Jack was a vigorous, active man until retirement. The not-O.K. feelings associated with retirement influenced Jack to withdraw. He kept to himself, paid no attention to his personal appearance, ate more, and exercised less. A 45-pound weight increase was followed by a serious heart attack. The term "retirement" is a negative, not-O.K. term. It says, "You are done; you're too old to work anymore; you're useless; lie down and die."

The gaining of excessive weight is a display of the depressed, get-away-from-it-all, I'm not O.K.–You're O.K. position.

It is indeed strange the difference a word makes. Individuals don't retire from high school; they have commencement exercises which say a new life phase is commencing. People don't retire from college; they have another commencement exercise or convocation which says another life phase is beginning. Why not a commencement from work which says a new productive phase is beginning? There are many active, useful, and productive activities which can be carried on for personal fulfillment or to serve society. Commencement is a "get on with it" word which says, "I'm still O.K. I'm a little older, a little more experienced, a little wiser, and I have the time to contribute to myself, to others, and to society."

Forcing active, productive people to stop work at 60 or 65 years of age is a waste of productive talent. More ridiculous are "retirement training programs" which emphasize Adult data such as pension rights, sick benefits, insurance, termination leave, and so on, and neglect the retiree's real problem, which is how to survive the change in life style. For most people, retirement is a psychological game with the retiree in the Victim's role. A work commencement program designed to deal with Parent and Child feelings and redirect productive activities at the new life phase makes more sense. Time structured around productive activities makes withdrawal, such as that in Jack's case, unnecessary. Fat fever seldom strikes the person who continues an active life after the formal work years are past.

Case

After 16 years with one firm, Horace was laid off owing to economic conditions. Unsuccessful in landing a new job quickly, he stopped trying and covered up by playing psychological games with his unsuspecting wife and withdrawing from family and friends. His pastimes included steady television gawking and playing solitaire accompanied by Cokes and snacks. Eventually Horace was recalled by his former employer and returned to work with an additional 30 pounds of blubber.

EXERCISE: REVIEWING MY ACTIVITIES

1. Make a list of your work and leisure-time activities (useful, productive projects and tasks).

Work	Leisure

2. Circle the activities which involve food and drink. Cross off items which are better described as pastimes, rituals, games, rackets, and withdrawal.

3. How can you decrease or eliminate food and drink from your activities?

4. Fat fever victims usually find it difficult to list leisure items which meet the productive, useful definition of activities. What hobbies, social or community projects, physical and recreational activities can you introduce to structure your leisure time more productively?

5. Can you relate your weight gain to a major change in your life, such as retirement, illness, unemployment, marriage, divorce, children going to school, children leaving home, death of a spouse or loved one, or other family or social change?

· How did you structure your time after the change?

· What effect did this have on your weight?

INTIMACY

Intimacy is a completely honest relationship with spontaneous expressions of love, caring, empathy, and appreciation. Intimacy is devoid of games, rackets, and rituals.

The pace of modern life and the fear of being rejected seem to be decreasing the amount of time structured around intimacy. The result is time structuring around games, rackets, rituals, pastimes, and withdrawal.

Significant parent figures, television, and movies provide a number of messages received by the little person in the Adapted Child. The adaptations stimulate receivers to structure life in ways which reduce intimacy. Some of these messages are:

· In general, people can't be trusted. Always expect another person to double-cross you at the first opportunity.

· Men are interested in women solely as sex objects.

· Women are bitchy, devious, and usually gold diggers.

· Girls are fair game and a boy's masculinity depends on how many "scores" he can make.

· Jews are too interested in money and Frenchmen too interested in sex. The English are cold, the Irish drink too much, and the Scots are tight. Blacks are lazy, Italians are gangsters, and so on and on.

· People with weak chins or eyes close together are not trustworthy.

Some people recognize these messages as prejudicial generalizations which are not supportable by fact. Unfortunately, most people accept at least some prejudicial messages as Adult data and use them as the rationale for decreased intimacy. On one hand is the message "Don't judge a book by its cover" while on the other is a set of prejudicial generalizations telling people to watch out for books with these covers.

Every mother shares real intimacy with a child who brings home a bouquet of wildflowers for Mommy. Every father shares real intimacy when his children charge out of the house screeching, "Daddy's home." Unfortunately, few people realize the long-term psychological value of intimacy and thus program their children in ways which reduce intimacy.

The pace of life and technological advances have reduced opportunities for intimacy. Watching television has replaced playing cards and other games as well as eliminated conversation. Front-porch sitting, which drew families and friends like a magnet, has disappeared. Saturday-night baths, in shared water in a tub on the kitchen floor, are a thing of the past. The automatic dishwasher has done away with the opportunity to talk while washing the dishes. The clothes dryer has eliminated the over-the-back-fence conversations while hanging the washing out to dry. The snowblower has eliminated the stop-for-a-rest conversations which we used to enjoy while shoveling. People seldom go for a stroll and stop to chat with neighbors. Anyone who is traveling on foot is jogging, which is hardly conducive to intimacy. The pollution of events and availability of transportation reduces the time family members spend together. Even central heating reduces intimacy; huddling around the kitchen stove on winter evenings was uncomfortable but was real sharing. Modern conveniences make the body comfortable but do little constructive for the mind.

• Kitchen-programmed people have a message that intimacy is related to food. Daddy's major stroking of mother is based on her cooking prowess. Charlie gets affectionate approval when he eats all his spinach and yelled at when he refuses to eat it. Eating more than a person wants or needs or eating food which is not liked is programmed on the assumption that the cook or hostess will be hurt if food is left. Intimacy means that a person should be comfortable sharing feelings about food or any other subject. Intimacy also means that the person is sensitive to another person's feelings but need not make unnecessary personal sacrifices.

• Bathroom-programmed people have a message that intimacy is related to the elimination of body waste or other impurities. Pottie perching or pimple picking is an intimate action. One young man said, "The only time I really felt close and intimate with my older sister was when she picked and squeezed the pimples and blackheads on my face and back. After a 9-year separation, I took my wife back to my home town to meet my sister for the first time. After two days of reminiscing, my sister said, "Your wife's a little dear. We all love her. I'm glad she has my old job of picking your back. It was evident that my sister also felt close while she was picking." Her comment indicated real acceptance of Marlie as a wife for her brother.

• Hurt-programmed people are devoid of intimacy. The desire for hostility and violence makes intimacy almost an impossibility. Making up after a fight is not intimacy. It is a form of trading in red stamps for a sexual encounter or some other prize. Hurts play so many games and participate in so many rituals and pastimes that there is little time or opportunity for intimacy.

• Love-programmed people structure a great deal of their time around intimacy. Displaying affection and being affectionate is a normal Love pattern. There is no underlying, phony reason for a Love's intimacy. Loves never say, "I love or like you because. . . . They skip the "because" and say, "I love you," or "I like you." The feelings of appreciation, empathy, affection, and general O.K.-ness which spill out of Love people are infectious. Love is the one infection worth catching.

Obese people have few opportunities for intimacy. Society frowns on obesity and some people cannot stand touching or socializing with a really fat person. Obese people do not like themselves, so it is not surprising that they give intimacy a low priority. The shortage of intimacy opportunities stimulates fat fever victims to structure time with games, rackets, pastimes, rituals, and withdrawal.

EXERCISE: TIME-STRUCTURING REVIEW

1. Based on your answers to the exercises on withdrawal, pastimes, rituals, games/rackets, activities, and intimacy, construct a personal time-structuring chart for your work life and your awake, leisure time. The example time-structuring chart is not good or bad but an example for direction only.

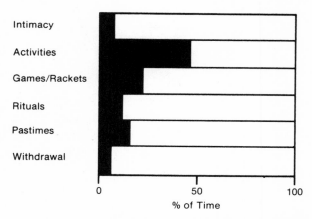

Example *How I Structure My Time*

		Intimacy		
		Activities		
		Games/Rackets		
		Rituals		
		Pastimes		
		Withdrawal		

How I Structure My Working Time   *How I Structure My Leisure Time*

2. What are the major differences between the structure of your work time and the structure of your leisure time? How do these differences influence fat fever?

3. List five things you will do to make changes which will decrease time spent on fat fever stimulators.

A.

B.

C.

D.

E.

CHAPTER
9
Redecision

You are fat because you decided to be fat. You can be slim if you decide to change the fat decision. By this time, you have an understanding of how fat fever is programmed through family patterns and how the fat fever program is perpetuated and passed on from generation to generation. This chapter provides additional insights and methods to assist you in investigating the basis of a redecision.

Redecision on fat fever does not normally require extensive reparenting, although obese persons who are seriously disturbed may need reparenting, through therapy, which is beyond the self-investigation and redecision described in this book.[1] The majority of fat fever sufferers can identify the elements of their own program and can do the spot [2] self-reparenting [3] necessary to change the program.

FICTION INPUT

Although much of a fat fever program is patterned by the big people around a young child, children receive other messages which are planted in the subconscious. Some beneficial and some destructive messages are passed on through nursery rhymes, fairy tales, myths, and fiction of all types. I shudder to think of the negative messages which some television programs inscribe on the subconscious minds of young children. A young child can be virtually destroyed for life when destructive, fictional messages reinforce an inappropriate family pattern.

Animism

A useful input to understanding a fat fever program can be gained by applying animism—the way myths explained life, primitive science, and the environment by applying a personality to objects and animals.

The morals contained in popular animistic stories are an influence on and an input to life programs. Consider the following examples:

1. *Impossible remedies are easily proposed, but not so easily carried through.* "The mice decided that a bell on the cat would give them a warning that the cat was coming. The wise old mouse said, 'That is a great idea, but who will bell the cat?' " Like the old mouse, fat fever sufferers know that there is a difference between proposing a remedy and carrying it through. Obese people have heard, "Use your willpower and you will lose weight," but they know it is far easier said than done. When fat fever is programmed in the subconscious, the program needs to surface before dieting can be successful.

2. *If you try to please everyone, no one will be pleased.* "A man and his son were walking beside their donkey on the way to market. Some men called them fools for walking. When the son rode, the men called him lazy for making his father walk. When the father rode, the men said, 'Shame, you ride while your poor little son walks.' When father and son both rode, the men berated them for overloading the poor beast. Finally, they tied the donkey to a pole and carried the donkey. The people laughed so much that the embarrassed father and son dropped the donkey into a creek where it drowned." Fat fever sufferers must realize that they cannot be Adapted Child pleasers. Some people are annoyed when you do not eat and some are annoyed when you eat too much. If you listen to everyone else, you will drown in blubber. Fat fever sufferers have to learn to please themselves and decide what is good for themselves first.

3. *Little by little does the trick.* "A thirsty crow found a pitcher with some water in the bottom. He dropped one pebble after another into the pitcher until it was full and the water

reached the top so that he could drink."Fat fever sufferers are programmed and gain excess weight over a lifetime, one pound at a time. Crash diets and starvation do not provide a lasting cure. Like the crow, the fat fever sufferer must use the Adult to solve the problem, analyze the fat fever program, and proceed toward objectives on a planned course, little by little, one step at a time.

4. *Vices are their own punishment.* "As punishment, Jupiter granted two neighbors, an avaricious man and an envious man, whatever each might wish for himself, on the condition that the neighbor got twice as much of each wish. The avaricious man wished for a pile of gold but was shattered when his neighbor got two piles. Not wishing his neighbor to have any joy, the envious man wished that one of his own eyes be plucked out, so that his neighbor would be struck blind." Fat fever sufferers must realize that the vices of gluttony and greediness and the resulting obesity are their own punishment which cannot be blamed on any other persons.

5. *It's useless to attack the unmovable.* "A snake slid into a blacksmith's shop where his skin was pricked by a sharp piece of iron. Time and time again in futility, the angry snake thrust his fangs at the unyielding iron until he gave up." Almost every obese person has felt the futility of attacking unyielding blubber. The angry Adapted Child cannot defeat obesity. Adult reasoning is the only road to success.

Fat fever sufferers can increase their understanding of their program by writing an animistic story describing themselves as the main character—an animal, bird, or some other animate object. Writing the story quickly allows the creative Child to identify the Kitchen program and to make Adult decisions on change.

Example: "Boris The Boar"

Boris the wild boar spent his days digging with his nose for succulent truffles. Although he did not often find sufficient truffles to satisfy his voracious appetite, he usually found enough other edibles on which to survive. During the year of the drought, food was in very short supply and a starving Boris joined a farmer's pig colony. Although the pig slop was not what Boris liked, he soon adapted to his environment. Boris became dependent very quickly and could no longer compete in the wilderness. He was destined to stay in the piggery, fully realizing that his fate was the slaughterhouse.

George, the creator of this animistic story, emigrated to Canada from Poland, where he had been a teacher. His first few years in Canada were difficult. His limited capability in English meant that he was often unemployed or employed as a low-paid laborer. While working on a farm, he met and married Tillie, the Kitchen-oriented farmer's daughter. George had not verbalized previously his concerns about dependency. As he shared his story, he said, "Boris and I are one. He is the largest pig in the piggery waiting for butchering. I'm butchering myself inside and outside."

George was withdrawingfrom life. Although he had mastered English and was relatively well educated, he continued laboring on his father-in-law's farm. He often stated his desire to secure a position where he could apply his education but put it off with one excuse after another. He had replaced his language albatross with an obesity albatross. It was easier for George to remain hidden on the farm than to take responsibility for his own life.

EXERCISE: ANIMISM

1. Write a short story describing yourself as an animal or bird or some other animate object.

2. Remain in the Adult and consider your animism carefully and explain:
A. Why you selected the animal, bird, or whatever.

B. What messages you get from your story.

3. Most young people dream often about a particular animal or vegetable. This animal is their totem.[4] Although the dream content may change, the totem usually appears in some form. Females dream about cats, horses, birds, reptiles, farm animals, flowers, and kitchen vegetables. Males dream about dogs, powerful horses, wild animals such as tigers, lions, wolves, large reptiles, and trees. The totem usually stops appearing in the early teens, but many fat fever sufferers report that their old totem or a new recurring totem reappears as their feeling of being overwhelmed by obesity increases. In her youth, Cora dreamed that she was always looking over her shoulder at grabbing hands. Just as she was about to be captured, she would turn into a beautiful bluebird and fly away to safety. The totem disappeared for 14 years, during which time she was happily married and secure. The totem-bluebird escape dream re-emerged at the time Cora gave up hope of defeating obesity. The totem stayed around during Cora's self-reprogramming, but she seldom sees it now. Self-responsibility and control negated Cora's need for the escape-hatch bluebird.

• Describe your totem dream and what it meant to you.

• Do you have a totem in your dream now? Is it the same one or a different totem? What does it mean?

• What similarities are there between your totem and your animistic story in question 1?

• Rewrite your animistic story with your totem as the main character.

• What new insight do you get about yourself?

4. Many of the sayings or morals used by a family and passed from generation to generation originated in animistic myths. The family sayings and messages from the stories become part of the young child's subconscious program. The list of morals which follow was developed from the animistic stories I read to my children plus sayings used in our family. Select three of these messages or use ones popular in your family and comment on their input to family patterns.
    • Gratitude and greed are enemies.
    • Beans in peace are better than a feast in fear.
    • Birds of a feather flock together.
    • Speak of the angels and they flutter their wings.
    • The seeds of evil grow to destroy you.
    • Fine feathers don't make a peacock.
    • Don't judge a book by its cover.
    • Conceit and destruction are bedmates.
    • Familiarity breeds contempt.
    • It is not hard to represent things as we wish them to be.
    • Give in to everyone and you will soon have nothing left to give.
    • Honesty is the best policy.
    • The strong and the weak cannot be friends.
    • A bird in the hand is worth two in the bush.
    • Greed often overreaches itself.
    • God helps them who help themselves.
    • Opportunity knocks only once and not with a hammer.
    • Curiosity killed the cat; satisfaction brought him back.
    • A stitch in time saves nine.

- Waste not, want not.
- One cannot escape his fate.
- Don't count your chickens before they're hatched.
- When you get two ends to meet, someone always moves the middle.
- Don't do as I do, do as I say.
- Experience is the best teacher.

A. Moral _____

B. Moral _____

C. Moral _____

5. What redecision action can you take to defuse the inappropriate messages programmed in question 3 above?

6. Describe yourself as a rock, barn, automobile, piece of furniture, tool, or other inanimate object which you perceive to have negative connotations.

7. Describe yourself as another inanimate object which you perceive to have positive connotations.

8. What redecisions must you make to change from the negative animism in question 6 to the positive animism in question 7.

Phony Dramas

Many people play out, in real life, the dramas in fairy tales, bedtime stories, mythology, folklore, nursery rhymes, movies, television, or other fiction. They adopt the Persecutor, Victim, or Rescuer roles and although the moves may be slightly different, the final outcome is similar to the outcome of the fictitious story.

It is beneficial to identity the fictitious drama or script which a person is following. Only by knowing the plot can a fat fever sufferer make changes in line with a cure.

Little Miss Muffet

Do you know a slender Little Miss Muffet who is turned off eating by minor disruptions? She is programmed to fear obesity and uses emotional and physical disruptions to reduce her intake of food. On the other hand, Big Miss Muffet uses emotional and physical disruptions as a reason to eat more. When the spider sits down beside her, she may run in fright but she always takes her curds and whey with her.

Aladdin's Lamp

Do you know a rotund Adapted Child Aladdin who sits around rubbing his hands, burning candles in church, or wishing on a good-luck charm for a spirit to appear and wipe away years of fat? There are no magic remedies or easy cures. Fat fever sufferers do not own Aladdin's lamp.

Old Mother Hubbard

Do you know an Old Mother Hubbard who is driven by a Helping Parent desire to push food onto the people around her whether or not they want or need it? Old Mother Hubbard works so diligently at her provider function that she programs obesity in her family. She is shattered when she eventually finds out that her family members can think and do for themselves without her continual pressure to "eat and you'll feel better." Old Mother Hubbard may be a thin Kitchen person because her meager resources, symbolized by the bare cupboard, cause her to deprive herself to provide for all those poor dogs around her.

Old King Cole

Do you know an Adapted Child Old King Cole who plays "Jolly Fat Fred"? He sits for hours watching television, his fat stomach resting on his knees, while he yells for his pipe and his bowl—of popcorn, that is, not to mention his beer. Although he is really sad, Old King Cole knows society expects jolliness from him. Having his Helping Parent wife Queenie as a built-in servant makes obesity bearable for Old King Cole.

Old Woman Who Lives in a Shoe

Do you know a woman who plays "Get The World Off My Shoulders"? She has so many pressures that she doesn't know what to do and gets her relief through initiating Hurt pattern activities. "She whipped them all soundly and put them to bed."

Little Jack Horner

Do you know an Adapted Child Little Jack Horner who eats up everything on his plate and expects recognition for eating up? If recognition is not provided by some other person, Little Jack Horner strokes himself, "What a good boy am I." The Jack Horners of our world are Kitchen-oriented and obese or potential candidates for obesity.

Ding Dong Bell

Do you know a Little Johnny Green who goes out of his way to destroy and hurt those who cannot fight back? Johnny's programmed, egocentric Hurt pattern says, "Throw pussy in the well." Do you know the Helping Parent/Rescuer, Little Tommy Stout, who always "pulls her out"?

The Queen of Hearts

Do you know a Love/Kitchen-oriented Queen of Hearts who invites a diet-busting game by making and displaying delicious, tempting food? Do you know the Knave of Hearts who plays "Midnight Marauder" and raids the pantry? Do you know the

Hurt-oriented King of Hearts who berates or beats the Knave for breaking the diet? Have you ever seen the Rescuer Queen of Hearts intervene to save the Knave from further punishment? This nursery rhyme is an example of a fat fever game played in many families and which contains all the game elements:

- Invitation to play.
- Plausible-appearing transactions.
- A hidden message.
- Persecutor, Victim, Rescuer roles.
- Role switches.
- A negative payoff.

Little Tommy Tucker

Do you know an Adapted Child Little Tommy Tucker who is programmed to be pleasant and good and is rewarded with junk food? Paying off Little Tommy Tucker, for his song, with obesity-inducing food is a Kitchen pattern. Who hasn't heard mother say, "If you're good until I finish my floor, I'll give you some candy." Kitchen-oriented people often bribe with food.

Jack Spratt Could Eat No Fat

Do you know a slender Adult Jack Spratt who eats sensibly and an obese Adapted Child Jacqueline Spratt who eats junk foods? Jack eats lean and Jacqueline eats fat until the platter is licked clean. Jacqueline piles on the blubber and says, "I know I shouldn't eat so much, but Jack eats so little and I can't waste food." Jacqueline's game is "If It Weren't For You."

The Three Bears

Do you know a Kitchen-oriented Goldilocks who plays "Nellie The Nibbler" and nibbles off all the plates yet can still clean up one plate? The dieting nibbler is found out eventually and runs away from life in the same way that Goldilocks ran away from The Three Bears.

Chicken Little

Do you know an obese Adapted Child Chicken Little who travels with other fat people, procrastinating about a diet until she is devoured by obesity? Overweight people are like Chicken Little who was hit on the head by an acorn and started out to tell the King that the sky was falling. Chicken Little was joined by Henny Penny, Ducky Lucky, Cocky Locky, Goosey Loosey, and Turkey Lurkey. The "birds of a feather flocked together" and met Foxy Woxy who used his Little Professor to manipulate the end of the story. It is only a matter of time before people hit on the head by obesity will join other overweight people who reinforce tragic life plans or scripts.

Hansel and Gretel

Do you know a Hansel or a Gretel who is continuously tempted by food which is left around by a phony Helping Parent with an ulterior motive, namely, fat children don't leave home? Controlling Parent witches are manipulating their children into a disaster much as the witch tempted Hansel and Gretel with a house made of sweets and then fattened Hansel for the oven. Unfortunately, only the rare strong-minded child will rebel as Hansel did.

The Ugly Duckling

Do you know an Ugly Duckling who continually heard, "Don't worry, you'll soon lose your baby fat," but never emerged as the beautiful swan? Children are born free and beautiful until they are programmed to be fat. Once obesity gets a good hold, it becomes a way of life until all hope disappears. Fat fever sufferers can change their programs until, like the Ugly Duckling, they emerge as sleek, graceful swans.

Rip Van Winkle

Do you know a Rip Van Winkle who slept in a cocoon of fat for 20 years and was shattered when he had to come out in the world again? Do you know a fat, sloppy Rip Van Winkle who has a son who is a precise, fat, sloppy copy of the father? Obese, Kitchen-oriented people unknowingly develop their children in their pattern. "Like father, like son" is more truth than fiction in the Kitchen family.

Rapunzel

Do you know a beautiful Rapunzel who has been encased in a tower of fat? Each time she tries to escape from obesity, her jailer cuts off her diet escape route much as the enchantress cut Rapunzel's hair. When she meets her prince charming, he is never good enough for our girl. Some parents and some husbands play "Chastity Belt" with the beautiful Rapunzel so that she can never let down her hair to the Rescuer.

Sleeping Beauty

Do you know a Sleeping Beauty who is waiting for a prince charming to save her from obesity? Do you know a fat frog who is waiting for a rescuing kiss from the beautiful princess? Many obese people sit around and wait for a Rescuer—a new diet, a stomach bypass, a Gray-Coated Savior, a new drug, or whatever. There is no external rescue available to most obese people. You have to be your own prince charming or kissing princess.

Beauty and the Beast

Do you know a beautiful woman who expects to save her obese mate only to find out that the Beauty-and-the-Beast routine doesn't work? Some Helping Parent/Rescuers believe that they can change an obese person from a fat frog into a handsome stallion but become frustrated and disenchanted with the lack of progress. Beauty seldom cures the Beast, whether it is a Hurt program, alcoholism, dishonesty, laziness, obesity, or any other character-related deficiency. If the Beast doesn't take responsibility for the change, it will never happen. There is a greater probability that Beauty will join the Beast in obesity than that the Beast will be rescued from fat fever.

Sisyphus

Do you know an obese Sisyphus who is always starting a new diet? Sisyphus is a character from Greek mythology who was destined to roll a large stone up a hill, only to have it roll back again as he got to the top, and he had to start over. The fat Sisyphus tries and tries but always ends up where he started. He is condemned to a lifetime cycle of dieting, nearly achieving success, then failing utterly. His Controlling Parent injunction is "Don't make it," but his Helping Parent says, "If you don't make it, try and try again."

Pinocchio

Do you know a Little Professor Pinocchio whose plot backfired? Pinocchio lied and lied about the location of the gold coins and was punished by having his nose get longer and longer with each lie. The real-life Pinocchio pretends to diet and lies and lies about the quantity, type, and frequency of food consumption. He is punished with a stomach which gets larger and larger.

EXERCISE: IDENTIFYING YOUR FICTIONAL MODEL

1. A change of your program is more comfortable once you have identified the fictitious characters who appear to be your subconscious models. List three fictitious characters from children's stories, mythology, folklore, comics, or other fiction who display elements of your program and family pattern. Explain your reason for choosing them.

My Model	Reason for Choice
A.	
B.	
C.	

2. Select a story theme which appears to fit your life pattern. Your theme may come from nursery rhymes, fairy tales, folklore, legends, mythology, and children's stories. The following stories, used in training sessions, may assist you in recalling the themes.

"Aladdin's Lamp"
"Ali Baba and the
        Forty Thieves"
"The Emperor's New Clothes"
"Dick Whittington's Cat"
The Swiss Family Robinson
"Little Red Riding Hood"
"Robin Hood"
"King Midas"
Tales of King Arthur
Tom Sawyer
"The Pied Piper"
"Sleeping Beauty"
"Jack and the Beanstalk"
"Puss in Boots"
"Chick, Chick, Halfchick"
"The Hare and the Tortoise"
"The Dog in the Manger"
"The Dog and the Shadow"
Alice in Wonderland

"Johnny Appleseed"
"Joe Magarac"
Gulliver's Travels
Don Quixote
Black Beauty
Little Women
"Cinderella"
"Snow White"
"Rumpelstiltskin"
"The Golden Goose"
"The Goose Girl"
"The Three Little Pigs"
"The Lion and the Mouse"
Tom Thumb
"The Tin Soldier"
"The Red Shoes"
*Rebecca of Sunnybrook
        Farm*
Pinocchio
Winnie the Pooh

Write a "Once upon a time" story, with yourself as the main character, which relates to the theme you have selected.

Theme _____

Once upon a time,

Analyze your story in the Adult. Can you identify any early decisions which you made about food, drink, and weight?

3. Rewrite your story (from question 2), changing the theme to one which will make a positive contribution to a continuing fat fever cure.

4. Who is the fictitious or real-life personality you most admire?

_____

Why?

• What examples or characteristics of this personality offer useful inputs for your redecision?

DREAMS

It is probable that this book and your responses to the exercises have stimulated you to dream about your childhood, parents, friends, family, life pattern, and so on. Some dreams are extensions of recent events while other dreams are dramas based on material hidden or camouflaged in the subconscious mind. Freud recognized that dreams contain insights into an individual's fears, desires, hopes, frustrations, and anxieties which are not always obvious or recognizable during waking hours. Dreaming does not just happen; it is a meaningful activity which fills a basic need to reduce the tension of living. Through dreams a person discharges the psychological tensions and impulses which are not expressed during waking hours.

Dreaming is a normal human function which happens to almost every person. Some people may dream more than others or at least have better dream recall. Individuals who say, "I never dream," should be saying, "I can't recall my dreams." Psychologists can recognize that a dream is probably in progress by the subject's pattern of eye movements. Persons who claim to be nondreamers often recall dreams when they are awakened during periods of REM (rapid eye movement).

The major hindrance to using dreams as a redecision input is that we have difficulty recalling our dreams. Under normal conditions, we recall only the dreams which happen just before we awaken or are in progress at the time of awakening. The method of awakening seems to have an effect on recall. When we wake up with a start, the dream is recalled, but when we wake up slowly and peacefully, recall is often blocked. Who hasn't said, "I had a crazy dream last night, but darned if I can remember what it was." Some people can even go back to sleep to finish a dream and still forget the dream.

Dreams are one outlet for some of the suppressed expressions of the personality. Although dreams may appear wild, weird, crazy, and distorted, they have a plot which has meaning in relation to recent events or to subconscious issues and concerns. In your dreams, you are freer to explore issues and areas which may be taboo during waking hours. Dream techniques may bring to the surface aspects of your personality, program, motivation, and life issues which have been blind spots to you.

The emotional upset from fat fever stimulates dreaming. Using transactional analysis to identify the psychological basis for a continuing cure is a further dream stimulation. Using dream content as input for program understanding and eventual redecision is beneficial. In short, dreams, no matter how crazy they may seem, reflect issues and motivations encountered in the waking hours. The dream content is an exploration of issues which is blocked when the dreamer is awake. The unpleasantness of the exploration may account for the inability of most people to recall a dream's content.

Dream analysis, which explains why we act in a certain way, requires the involvement of a professional therapist. The Gestalt technique, used here, emphasizes discovery of the dreamer's various selves in the dream and provides an opportunity for personal leveling about previously hidden or blocked messages.

Gestalt techniques reinforce the principle of self-responsibility. Dreams are useful input only if a fat fever sufferer is willing to accept responsibility for the input surfaced through the technique. On a number of occasions, group members have related recurring dreams (dreams which are repeated several times), only to withdraw, defensively, during the group discussion.

- We're making too much of this. Hell, it's only a dream.
- I can't accept that a crazy dream has meaning.
- I've been putting you on—I didn't dream that, I made it up. Ha ha ha ha.
- Role-play a garbage can. No dice; I may be fat but I'm not nuts.
- It scares me to think that the violence in my dreams may be the suppressed me. I'd rather let it drop. I don't want to know.

It is unreasonable to expect early acceptance and assumption of responsibility for disturbing or uncomfortable dream messages. Generally a person scales the Dreamer's Ladder step by step:

Step 1: Skepticism—Show and tell.
Step 2: Questioning—Is there meaning?
Step 3: Awareness—Understanding.
Step 4: Acceptance—Responsibility.

The message may be rejected immediately or at any step during the climb. The hierarchical climb, depicted on the model, may take minutes, hours, days, or weeks, depending on the participant's program, need for understanding, and desire to assume responsibility.

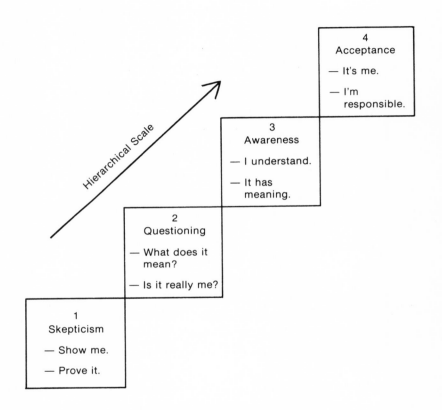

DREAMER'S LADDER

Case

Tara started eagerly but soon adopted a defensive posture about her dream content. The learning-group members listened silently and intently as Tara related her dream and played out the roles. As she progressed, her voice got louder and louder; it was evident that Tara was receiving some disturbing messages.

Finally, she stopped her role play and in a childlike voice blurted out, "I can't accept that; I'm not like that—that's too ugly a feeling for me. Anyway, it's only a dream. I'd like to drop it here."

Positive learning groups operate on the principle that participants decide what to do, when and how much to participate, and when to stop. There is no compulsion to participate in any exercise or discussion and no one who feels uncomfortable is forced to continue. Thus, in Tara's situation, the group moved on to another participant.

Later during the session Tara indicated step-1 skepticism: "I wish someone could show me, prove to me, that my dream has meaning for me." A group member suggested, "Maybe you'll get more insight by a safer involvement in my dream exercise. I'm not too comfortable in the show-and-tell role, but I need all the input I can get. I was just wondering though, if you got no input from your dream, maybe you could consider why it got you so upset?"

Six sessions later, Tara leveled with the group, announcing that she had scaled the Dreamer's Ladder. Her dream had a recurring theme in which she was competing in a number of competitive events but finished second each time. She had stopped her role play 6 weeks ago, when she was describing how she had let the sure dog-show winner, an Irish setter, out of his cage and out the door, where the dog was struck by a passing car. Tara explained, "I was upset about my envy racket for the second-place finishes but was more upset and disbelieving when I let the dog out to be killed. I love dogs. I'd never do anything to hurt a dog. Therefore it didn't make much sense to me to go on. I really do have an envy racket. I've never come first at anything. The few times I've had a chance to win, my sister Colleen has beat me out. I envy all the winners, and most of all I envy Colleen. I wondered about the dog, and although I hate to say it, Colleen is an Irish name and she has beautiful auburn hair. I envy Colleen but I wouldn't hurt a hair on her head; nevertheless, the dream is scary. I know I am responsible for my envy racket and I've contracted with myself to do some more racket busting. I know now that each time I am envious, I head for the refrigerator so I can kill two birds—envy and weight—with one stone."

The Gestalt dream technique introduced here is a simple method to determine some of the here-and-now tensions, frustrations, and anxieties which may be restricting a cure. The technique does not analyze *why;* it identifies and clarifies *how.* Dream consideration provides additional input and scope for redecision. Follow these steps:

1. Make written notes or use a recorder to register dream content immediately on awakening. Even a 5-minute delay is enough time to forget a dream. Record all the dream, people, places, objects, and actions down to the most minute detail you can recall.

2. Describe the dream in your own words in the order that it happened.

3. Using the first person "I," role-play each item, person, etc., in the dream.[5] Some therapists suggest that what appear to be the least emotional parts be roled-played first and the most emotional parts last. I find it more beneficial and realistic to role-play the parts in chronological order—that is, role-play the items in the order they appear in the dream.

4. Relate, force-fit if necessary, your dream content and role play to your ego states, strokes, discounts, injunctions, family patterns, games, rackets, life positions, and so on. Describing the dream events in transactional analysis terms provides a common language and a recipe for additional understanding. When the dream is considered in a group session, the group assists by open-ended questioning and limits direct interpretation. This allows the dreamer to interpret and assume responsibility and ownership for the results.

5. Identify the lessons or new insights arising from your dream technique and make a decision on corrective action.

Should you wish more detailed information on dream theory, you may wish to read Freud's *The Interpretation of Dreams* [6] and French and Fromm's *Dream Interpretation.*[7]

Case

Marion role-played a recurring dream in which she was in an elevator alone. Each time she reached out to push the stop button, the panel disappeared. When she pulled her hand back, the button panel reappeared. In between these wild, uncontrollable elevator rides, she would appear on a stage as a curvy go-go dancer. During her dance, Marion gained weight until the audience laughed and shouted out obscene and insulting remarks. When she could no longer stand the catcalls and put-downs, the scene shifted back to the elevator ride.

• At first Marion described the elevator as a Controlling Parent who would not let her get off and the disappearing panel as part of the Controlling Parent elevator. She recognized herself as the trapped Adapted Child.

• The dance was described and played out as a Free Child with the stage as a Helping Parent providing her the outlet to perform.

• The audience started out as the Free Child enjoyers but quickly changed to the criticizing Parent Persecutor.

• Marion saw the emerging fat as her Controlling Parent saying, "Quit play-acting. You're too fat to be a go-go dancer. Keep it up and everyone will laugh at you."

• The elevator on the second trip changed to the Helping Parent/Rescuer, shielding Victim Marion from the persecuting put-downs. Marion now saw the disappearing panel as her Little Professor manipulating the Drama so that she could stay in her protective cocoon.

• Being allowed to dance and perform was a form of warm stroke which was turned to cold and zigzag strokes because of obesity.

• Marion's injunctions were: "Don't be yourself, you're too fat to dance"; "Don't enjoy yourself, you should sit around and feel sorry"; "Don't give anyone a reason to laugh at you, hide out instead."

• Marion's game, "Jolly Fat Freda," was played out in her dream. Marion ended up with negative payoffs of put-downs and isolation, similar to the payoffs she received when awake.

• She identified her racket as inadequacy and her stamps as a black depression collection. Most elevators are bright pastel colors, but the black dream elevator symbolized her depression.

Marion saw herself as a basically fun-loving Free Child with a dominant Controlling Parent which restricted Free Child play. She loved to dance but seldom got a chance as few men search out an obese partner. She mentioned that at parties she often danced alone but stopped as soon as she felt that people were laughing at her. Playing "Jolly Fat Freda" fooled others, but she knew that her depression and feeling of inadequacy were real. Marion described the elevator as symbolizing her fat friends. They protected her, didn't make fun of her or put her down, but like the continuously moving elevator, they never stopped gaining weight. Marion said, "I know my first act is to get off the elevator; I can't stand the black, depressing walls. If I don't get off now I'll never make it."

EXERCISE: DREAMS

1. Describe one of your dreams as if it were happening now.

2. Imagine you are each person, each animal, or each object in your dream and, using the first person "I," act out each part in the order it appears in the dream. The dialogue between the various parts of your dream allows you to experience feelings and move rapidly from ego state to ego state. Feel free to move around and act out the roles in any way which feels comfortable to you. What ego state did you assign to each role?

Roles	Ego State (CP, HP, A, AC, FC, LP)

3. Describe and categorize, as warm, cold, and zigzag, the giving and receiving of the strokes which occur in the dream.

4. Are the strokes discounted in the dream?

5. What is the relationship between the dream strokes and your waking life? For example: do you stroke or receive strokes from the persons in your dream; do you give and receive similar strokes and discounts; are you stroke-deprived; do the dream strokes indicate any internal frustrations, fears, or anxieties?

6. Dreams often relate to programmed "don'ts" or injunctions. Does your dream reinforce your injunctions or does it go against the don'ts in your program?

7. Dreams are a type of drama, often with dream characters adopting the Rescuer, Victim, and Persecutor roles.
• Who or what took on each role in your dream?

• Describe the role switches.

• Who got the negative payoff?

• How does your dream relate to your real-life games? For example: are the dreams similar; are the characters and roles similar; have you gone through a similar drama in real life?

8. What new information has the dream exercise brought to the surface about you and your family pattern?

9. List three factors from your dream analysis which will be useful to you in altering your fat fever program.

A.

B.

C.

10

Activating a Cure

Most fat fever cases are self-curable once the patient accepts responsibility for the condition and makes an Adult decision to deal with the problem.

I am not suggesting that therapy is ineffective. Some unfortunate people have so many psychological issues intertwined with the fat fever condition that they require therapy. Also, it is easier and possibly faster to analyze your program and to activate a cure with effective, professional help. Unfortunately, therapy is both costly and time-consuming, and often a qualified transactional analyst is not practicing in a location convenient to the patient.[1]

At times in my transactional analysis workshops, I recognize someone who would benefit from therapy. Usually, the individual has come to the same conclusion but is blocked by the stigma of treatment. "What will my friends and family think when they find out that I am being treated by a shrink? I don't know whether I can stand the embarrassment."

Although the "in thing" with some people is to be in therapy, most people neglect needed therapy or keep secret the fact that they are receiving treatment. Therapy is an O.K. activity. A person who seeks therapy is taking responsibility. There is no reason to be embarrassed when you make a rational, logical decision to get professional help. Also, there is no reason to share the information that you are in treatment unless your feelings of embarrassment, shame, or inadequacy are counterproductive to a cure. Dealing with these feelings early on in therapy will be helpful.

I do not expect instant acceptance of therapy as an O.K. activity, although we are moving slowly in that direction. There are hundreds and possibly millions of people who need or would benefit from treatment, but the "What will people think?" message blocks them from seeking professional help.

Worrying about what other people think is an Adapted Child response. When mother says, "Wash your face and comb your hair, Auntie's coming," or "Weed the flower garden—what will the neighbors think?" the Adapted Child hears the message as, "You don't do things for yourself, you do things to please someone else." More appropriate messages would relate cleanliness to hygiene and health and weeding the flower garden to beauty for oneself first.

Throughout this book, redundancy has been used in an effort to accentuate the importance of the principle of self-responsibility. Self-cure without professional help is a practical goal for persons who are willing to assume total responsibility for their condition. Denial of personal responsibility is the fertilizer for growing obesity as well as other emotional or psychological problems. When a fat person does not take total personal responsibility for obesity, he or she attributes the causes of that obesity to some other person. If that other person accepts the responsibility, a "Blame" game is initiated.

"You persecuted me, so now I'm fat. Once we establish your responsibility, you can be my Rescuer. By blaming you, I can switch you to the Victim role. If I am skilled at the "See What You Made Me Do" game, I can keep the game going indefinitely. So long as you continue as my patsy and I can keep you feeling responsible for my obese condition, I am not compelled to exert any effort toward personal change. When my obesity gets too much to endure peacefully, I can cash my brown-stamp collection in on you, my patsy, in ways which will feed my fat fever as well as affect you physically and emotionally."

Complete acceptance of the following statements is a must before a self-cure can be activated:

· I am responsible for my feelings and behavior.

- I am responsible for my fat fever condition.
- No other person is responsible or to blame for my condition, feelings, or behavior.
- I can and will cure my case of fat fever.

If you are unwilling to accept complete responsibility for your condition or unable to understand that you and you alone hold the key to a permanent cure, you have no chance for a self-cure. You may as well throw this book into the closest trash can and resign yourself to obesity. If you have enough Adult logic to understand that the statements regarding responsibility are correct and completely true, then by all means continue reading: a permanent self-cure is practical and possible for you.

You can reinforce this most important factor by reviewing your answers to the *Understanding My Responsibility* exercise in Chapter 2.

CONTINUING THE INVESTIGATION

The material provided in this book plus the exercise responses are designed to stimulate self-awareness and responsibility. Of course, it is unreasonable to expect that you will have all the answers. As you proceed with activation of a self-cure program, a stream of additional information and insights will surface which will increase self-awareness. It is important that you continue searching for new inputs and understanding which reinforce and support the psychological and behavioral changes which you wish to make.

Investigation of your program is a search for answers to the following questions:

- Who and what am I?
- What am I really like?
- How did I get this way?
- Which parts of my program induced fat fever?
- What redecisions should I make for a continuing cure?

Quite often persons reviewing their program will say, "I see that as a reasonable deduction, but how can I be sure about the meaning?" Of course, there is no way that we can be 100 percent sure about meanings, but the transactional analysis concepts are so interrelated that the data retrieved through the different concepts have a consistency which is difficult to refute. It is these supportive and reinforcing relationships which make transactional analysis a useful self-analysis and self-cure tool. One does not need to be a therapist to understand and to react to the recurring messages which pop out of the exercise responses.

The ideas, concepts, and techniques which follow are additional helpful inputs for a continuing investigation.

Program Questionnaire

Transactional analysts use a life-script process which combines a questionnaire and interview designed to provide insights or to raise questions about a patient's life program or pattern. The *My Program* exercise is a short version of the process which is appropriate for investigating a fat fever script.[2] The questions are designed to review your previous exercise responses and to assist you in completing your self-contract.

EXERCISE: MY PROGRAM

Answer the following questions carefully. After you have completed them, go back over each item and reexamine it thoroughly to surface additional data. Finally, circle the items where you got new insights.

1. Describe yourself.

2. What do you like and dislike most about yourself?

3. How long have you had fat fever?

4. How many times have you tried dieting?

5. Why did your diets fail?

6. What bad feelings do you have about yourself?

7. When did you first feel these bad feelings?

8. What do you consider to be your greatest weakness? Why?

9. What was your favorite children's story?

10. What part of the story did you like best?

11. What was your totem? Does it still appear in your dreams?

12. What are your dreams like generally?

13. Do you have a recurring dream? Describe the theme.

14. What do you want most out of life?

15. When will you die?

16. What inscription will be on your tombstone?

17. What is your most serious problem?

18. Do you often feel that something, whether physical or psychological, is wrong with you?

19. How do you structure your time?

20. What was/is your nickname(s)? Why?

21. Describe your closest friend.

22. Describe your spouse and children.

23. Describe your mother.

24. What did your mother say about food?

eating?

weight?

25. How did your mother criticize you?

compliment you?

26. What was/is your mother's favorite
ego state?
racket?
stamp?
game?
injunction?
stroke?
ritual?
activity?
pastime?
advice?
saying?

27. What was/is your mother's primary and secondary family pattern?

28. Describe your father.

29. What did your father say about
food?

eating?

weight?

30. How did your father
criticize you?

compliment you?

31. What was/is your father's favorite
ego state?
racket?
stamp?
game?
injunction?
stroke?
ritual?
activity?
pastime?
advice?
saying?
32. What was/is your father's primary and secondary family pattern?

SELF-REPARENTING

Every individual has some Parent messages which are O.K. and other Parent messages which are not O.K. It is difficult or at least uncomfortable for most people to recognize the negative inputs from natural parents. When we talk about our parents, we are often blocked by the "beautiful Mommy" and "wonderful Daddy" syndrome which is distorted by time. By now you should have come to the conclusion that your parents were human, with many good qualities and some imperfections.

Self-reparenting is an Adult activity. After analyzing collected data, the individual makes a rational, independent decision on the positive and negative parental inputs which stimulate fat fever. Remaining in the Adult allows an individual to determine what inputs will be kept and what inputs will be eliminated or at least controlled. The individual creates a new Parent ego state which incorporates the O.K. parts of the present Parent and replaces the not-O.K. parts with messages which support a cure.[3]

The question of total reparenting versus spot reparenting at one level is an academic argument so far as fat fever is concerned. A fat fever sufferer requires reparenting which eliminates or at least defuses the messages which are causing obesity. A person can use the Adult to spot self-reparent at one level, but total reparenting is a task for a qualified therapist.

How To Self-Reparent

1. A good knowledge of transactional analysis is necessary for effective self-reparenting. This book provides sufficient input for the average person, but if you wish more detailed transactional analysis material, other effective sources are listed in the Bibliography. Attendance at a transactional analysis workshop can be an exciting and beneficial personal-growth experience.

2. An output of your exercise responses is the realization that the negative parental inputs need to be eliminated, defused, or replaced. Individuals give themselves Permission to make

necessary changes without feeling hurt or uncomfortable use the Adult to reason out the issues, thus providing themselves the Protection of knowing that the right action is being taken and by investigation and continued learning provide themselves the Potency to carry through with self-reparenting.[4]

3. The exercises in Chapter 3 and the *Parent* exercises in Chapter 4 are provided to assist you in getting to know your significant parental figures. It is recommended that you review your responses to these exercises and make any corrections or additions which you consider appropriate. You must know your Parent well before you can activate self-reparenting. Should you want further input on parents, I recommend Muriel James's *What Do You Do with Them Now That You've Got Them?* [5]

4. The *Child* and *Adult* exercises in Chapter 4 are provided to assist you in determining the input of the Adult and Child to fat fever and to identify how your Adult and Child is contaminating your Parent. Often we may be acting Parent with the input coming from the Adult or the Child. At other times, the input comes from our Parent ego state. When a person is considering reparenting it is important to realize that all ego states can energize parental-appearing behavior.

In self-reparenting your Adult communicates with your Adapted Child, your Free Child, and your Little Professor to determine what the Child needs to cure fat fever. The Adapted Child may need Adult Permission to turn off the parental orders to "Eat up and don't waste food." The Free Child may need Adult reinforcement that it is O.K. to be intimate and enjoy yourself without food or drink. The Little Professor may need Adult input which identifies and defuses the psychological hooks and ulterior messages which are initiating fat fever games.

5. The input from transactional analysis plus the data collected in the exercises are considered in the Adult. The Adult now knows what is good and not so good about the Parent and contracts to practice the new Parent activities. For a period of time, activating new Parent behaviors will be difficult and require a considerable effort, but eventually the new Parent will take over and become an integral part of the Parent.[6] Patience is

the fourth "P" (after Permission, Protection, and Potency) required for reparenting.

EXERCISE: SELF-REPARENTING

1. Make a list of five positive and five negative food-, drink-, and weight-related messages which are part of your Parent ego state. Reviewing your answers to the *Parent* exercises in Chapter 4 and the exercises in Chapter 9 will be helpful. It may also help you to recall how your parents behaved at mealtimes with regard to habits, mannerisms, eating rituals, formality or informality, conversation, rules, force, and fun.

	Positive	Negative
1		
2		
3		
4		
5		

2. Self-reparenting means that you give yourself Permission to replace the negative tapes with messages which will support a fat fever cure. You have assumed complete responsi-

bility for your condition and have developed a knowledge of transactional analysis and collected data which combine to afford you the Protection and Potency necessary for reparenting. How can you defuse and replace the negative messages?

3. Sit back quietly and close your eyes. Imagine you are at a reception at a first-rate hotel. For weeks you have been watching what you eat and have lost 7 pounds. The buffet dinner is beautiful and contains all the foods you like most. What conversation is going on in your head among your Parent, Adult, and Child?

Which ego state wins? What is the outcome?

4. Sit down in a quiet place and think about your fat fever condition. Initiate an internal dialogue between your Adult and Child to determine what your Adopted Child, Free Child, and Little Professor need to cope with fat fever.

5. Initiate an internal dialogue between your Adult and Parent to determine what changes you need to make in your Helping Parent and Controlling Parent to facilitate a fat fever cure.

Internal Dialogues

The internal-dialogue approach introduced in the self-reparenting exercise above is a useful technique to continue as you progress toward a permanent cure. Continuing on with the Adult-to-Child or Adult-to-Parent internal dialogue decreases the possibilities of being hooked by the Adapted Child decisions made when you were very little and the Parent beliefs and Child distortions which are contaminating your rational, logical Adult.

CLEANING UP THE ADULT

A fat fever cure requires the removal of messages accepted in the Adult which are based on Parent beliefs and Child distortions. This condition is described as *contamination.*

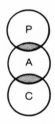

The Adult treats contaminated

messages as fact and uses the

input as the basis for action.

Defusing and replacing negative parts of the Parent need to be combined with the decontamination of the Adult. The decision to take responsibility for your condition means that you are also ready and willing to think and feel for yourself.

Transactional analysis is based on the self-control assumptions that you can learn to:

- Think for yourself.
- Trust yourself.
- Make your own decisions.
- Express your own feelings.

The contaminated messages in your Adult are not yours. They belong to someone else who programmed you long ago. If you accept and agree with the basic transactional analysis assumptions about self-control, you are ready to clean up your Adult.

EXERCISE: CLEANING UP THE ADULT

On the basis of your recall and a review of your answers to the contamination exercise in Chapter 4 (see page 80), prepare a list of five messages about food, drink, weight, and physical activity which are Adult contaminations. How and from whom did the messages originate? How do you know now that the messages are Child distortion or Parent beliefs and not supportable by fact?

	Contaminated Messages	How Originated and from Whom?	How I Know They Are Not Factual
1.			
2.			
3.			
4.			
5.			

CHANGING THE PATTERN

The thesis of this book is that a person's obese or nonobese condition is programmed in early childhood. The primary and secondary family patterns, described in Chapter 3, say "Be fat!" or "Don't be fat!" Some fortunate individuals are saved from obesity by their physiology or by an active Adult which is able to defuse the program. In most cases, it is more a matter of luck than good management which keeps one person in a Kitchen family slender while the other members progress to obese conditions. A person programmed to fat fever has a 99 percent probability of getting the disease sooner or later. Sometime fat fever doesn't strike until a person is past 30 or 40 years of age, but one thing is sure: if the program says "Be fat!" you will gain weight eventually unless you make an Adult decision to change your program.

The family program pressures a person to make early decisions about food, drink, and weight. These premature decisions are self-destructive. Action toward a cure requires that patients bring to the surface the underlying foundation of the family program and change the program based on here-and-now realities.

EXERCISE: REVIEWING MY FAMILY PATTERN

1. Based on a review of your responses to the *Family Pattern* exercises in Chapter 3, develop a list of positive words and phrases and a list of negative words and phrases which describe your primary and secondary family patterns.

My Primary Pattern Is _____		My Secondary Pattern Is _____	
Positive Words/Phrases	Negative Words/Phrases	Positive Words/Phrases	Negative Words/Phrases

2. Circle the words which are stimulants of fat fever. Take each word at a time and have an internal dialogue between your Adult and Parent and your Adult and Child to bring to the surface the full effect of the message on your program.

3. List five Adult decisions which will defuse the fat-inducing messages from your family pattern.

A.

B.

C.

D.

E.

Changing a program is made difficult by the blockage most people have about seeing their natural parents clearly. The task is made easier when you accept the idea that identifying negative parental inputs does not include blaming your parents. Most parents do what they think is right for their children at the time.

Parents have internal and external pressures which stimulate them to act in specific ways. Sometimes these actions leave a positive message and sometimes they leave a negative scar. Accepting this condition as normal and attaching no blame provide the Permission to change or defuse any tapes which are inducing fat fever.

In my own case, I found it very difficult to reduce my parents to a size with which I could cope comfortably. My father died when I was 7 and my mother worked very hard to raise three children. Each time I tried to collect data on my father, I ended up with a long list of positive characteristics and no negatives. In actual fact, I was describing a fantasy father who had been created in my mind by my mother's stories and my own young boy's need for a perfect father in heaven.

Each time I tried to analyze my mother, I ended up with a similar situation—all positives and no negatives. It was imposs-ible for me to get past the love and devotion she displayed by working at menial tasks to raise a family alone. I remembered the time when I looked at her through the kitchen window and saw the few pennies on the table and the tears of despair on her face. When I ran in to see why she was crying, she protected me from reality by saying, "I dropped a piece of firewood on my foot and it brought the tears to my eyes. I'll be all right in a minute or so." I remembered how she walked miles to work in the cold Ottawa winters, to save the streetcar fare so that we could have a toy at Christmas.

I pictured my mother as a martyr, a savior, and an angel of mercy. I know that she was a wonderful mother in my childhood as she was an available, understanding friend in my young adult life, and at 76 she is still an energetic, independent, warm-stroke supporter of my every endeavor.

I used transactional analysis and the exercises in this book to unblock my recall. Now I see my mother in more objective terms. I see her as a person with all the normal strengths and weaknesses. I know the positive messages which stimulated me to success and personal growth and I know the negative messages from the secondary Kitchen program which influenced fat fever. Knowing all this has made me closer to my mother. I see her now as a complete person, not as a character from a fairy tale or a prayer book. The unblocking has caused my love for my mother to go deeper than before because now I really under-stand and appreciate her as a person, not as an angel.

EXERCISE: UNBLOCKING MY PROGRAM

1. If your family pet could talk, how would it describe your father, your mother, and your family pattern? It will be easier if you imagine yourself as the family pet.

Father

Mother

Family pattern

2. Imagine yourself as a little child sitting underneath the dining-room table listening to a conversation on food and weight between your mother and father. Write out their conversation.

3. Imagine your parents as children.
What is your mother's little-girl reaction to food and weight?

What is your father's little-boy reaction to food and weight?

4. Respond to the following questions based on your answers to questions 1 to 3 above.
A. What new insights did you get about your mother?

your father?

your primary and secondary family patterns?

yourself?

B. Are you acting on negative messages?

C. Are you passing on the negative messages to your children?

D. What are you thinking at this moment?

SELF-CONTRACT

A self-contract is an agreement with yourself that you will take specific cure-related actions. You need to decide:
- What changes you want to make.
- How you can make the changes.
- How to measure the changes as you progress.
- What the consequences of the change will be.
- How any other persons will be affected.

Therapists use contracts with patients to establish a be- havioral change objective and to reinforce the change until it becomes a natural rather than a forced or calculated reaction. Often the therapy contract is written out, and at times it is signed by the therapist and the patient.

A self-contract is similar but is structured by the individual concerned. At times, a person may be involved in a transactional analysis learning group and get help from other participants or share a contract with them. Sharing is useful, supportive, and reinforcing behavior but is not essential. No one has to see or be involved in your self-contract unless you wish. Accepting responsibility means that you can write your contract and get on with your cure.

The exercises in this book are designed to gather data and to increase understanding. Reviewing your responses will assist you to develop a self-contract for a continuing cure.

EXERCISE: MY CONTRACT

1. I contract with myself to cure my case of fat fever, permanently.

2. I accept complete responsibility for my condition.

3. My measurable objectives and time schedule are (review the *Weight Objectives* exercise in Chapter 2):

Elements	Present Condition	Milestone Objectives					
		3 Months	6 Months	9 Months	12 Months	15 Months	18 Months
Weight (lbs.)							
Condition Category							
Body Measures Waist Hips Chest Buttocks Other							

4. Other measurable changes which I will make are (review the *Symptom Awareness* exercise in Chapter 2):

Eating speed _____

Times eat daily _____

Reasons for eating _____

Calorie intake daily _____

Physical activity _____

Other _____

5. I contract to make the following changes in my program: (It is not necessary to make entries beside each factor. Only make entries on behaviors or feelings in which you perceive a need for change, behaviors which you can change, and behaviors which you want to change.)

A. Changes in my stroking pattern (review Chapter 3).

B. Changes in my family pattern (review Chapter 3).

C. Changes in my subpersonalities (review Chapter 4).
   Controlling Parent

   Helping Parent

   Adapted Child

   Free Child

Little Professor

Contaminated Adult

D. Changes in my communication pattern (review Chapter 5).

E. Changes in playing my Drama roles (review Chapters 6, 7, and 9).

F. Changes in my life positions as they relate to fat fever (review Chapter 6).

G. Changes in my (review Chapter 6):
Rackets

Stamp Collections

H. Changes in my fat fever games (review Chapters 7 and 9).

I. Changes in my time structuring (review Chapter 8): Withdrawal

Rituals

Activities

Pastimes

Games/Rackets

Intimacy

6. I will recycle and review this material at least quarterly until I am sure that my cure is permanent.

_____   _____
Date   Initials

RECYCLE AND REVIEW

By this time you have made a number of new decisions about

your family pattern and fat fever program. For some time to come, you will have to consciously activate the decision until it becomes a natural feeling, emotion, and action.

Disrupting your old program will probably free a considerable amount of time. The natural temptation is to fill up the time with games, rackets, rituals, and pastimes. An ongoing change in a program and a permanent cure require that the individual practice and consolidate the new skills and techniques. It is not enough to say, "I understand my problem and I know what I have to do." It takes a continuing, conscious effort to carry it off.

There is little doubt that you can and will lose weight if you change your fat fever program. That in itself is not enough. When obese people lose weight and eventually reach their target, they are hung up with the fear of gaining back their excess pounds. If you stick to your relearning, you will not gain weight; but if you revert to your old program, which is still tugging at you, you will be back to square one very soon. The most important thing you must learn is to be O.K. for yourself. Stop thinking fat. Think thin. It's a great feeling.

I recommend that you review the material in this book, your responses to the exercises, and your contract at least every 3 months until you are satisfied that you are in complete control. As new information surfaces, revise or add to your answers. It is beneficial to practice internal dialogue, dream techniques, and the other techniques as part of a continuing investigation, review, and recycle.

A permanent fat fever cure takes time and effort. Review and recycle is a necessary step. If you really want to be O.K., you will not neglect this important part of the process.

CHAPTER
11
Epilogue

I hesitate to call this a conclusion. The information in this book is the framework for a beginning. It doesn't end here. Fat fever will not disappear magically when you close the book's cover. A fat fever cure takes continuing emotional and physical commitment and involvement as you progress toward the objectives established in your self-contract.

Millions of obese people are living less than the full lives which they deserve and desire as they move steadily and surely toward serious illness and premature death. People are not robots or dumb animals. Give yourself Permission to think for yourself, to redecide your program, and to make the emotional and behavioral changes which energize a continuing cure. Decide here and now to dance through life rather than waddle uncomfortably along.

Obese people have a defeatist attitude. Time and time again I hear, "I've tried everything and nothing works for me." Transactional analysis will work if you accept full responsibility for your feelings and actions. Remember Edgar A. Guest's lines:

> Just start in to sing as you tackle the thing
> That "cannot be done" and you'll do it.[1]

Every person has the right to a full, joyful, and productive life. I am dismayed to see so many people destroyed by fat fever—a curable disease.

Good luck with your reprogramming.

FRANK LAVERTY
Ottawa, Canada, 1977

REFERENCES AND FOOTNOTES

Chapter 1

1 The credit for the initial development of transactional analysis goes to Dr. Eric Berne and the participants in the San Francisco Transactional Analysis Seminar. Their work has been extended and enlarged by the thousands of interested members of the International Transactional Analysis Association. The evolvement of TA as a public language makes it impractical to footnote each term or concept, and therefore general credits only are provided although I fully realize that others may have enlarged on the concept.

2 Eric Berne, *What Do You Say After You Say Hello?* (New York: Grove Press, 1972), chap. 3.

3 Claude Steiner, *Scripts People Live: Transactional Analysis of Life Scripts* (New York: Grove Press, 1974), chap. 14.

4 A Glossary containing special terms is provided on page 232. A Bibliography with recommended readings is provided on page 236.

Chapter 2

1 The principle of self-responsibility is basic to TA and has been mentioned by other authors. An excellent description of the principle was included in Dr. Charles Stewart's newsletter, "The Way We Are—Who Promised You The Rose Garden," published by C.D. Stewart Assoc. Inc., West Tower, Center Square, 1500 Market St., Philadelphia, Pa.

Chapter 3

1 Muriel James and Dorothy Jongeward, *Born To Win* (Reading, Mass.: Addison-Wesley, 1971), chap. 3, provides a detailed description of stroking.

2 Eric Berne, *What Do You Say After You Say Hello?* (New York: Grove Press, 1972), chap. 8, describes family culture in relation to sphincters.

Chapter 4

1 Muriel James and Dorothy Jongeward's *Born To Win* (Reading, Mass.: Addison-Wesley, 1971), chaps. 5, 6, and 9, contains a comprehensive description of the ego states and the six subpersonalities.

Chapter 5

1 Eric Berne, *What Do You Say After You Say Hello?* (New York: Grove Press, 1972), chap. 2.
2 Alvyn Freed, *TA for Tots* (Sacramento, Calif.: Jalmar Press, 1973), and *TA for Kids* (Sacramento, Calif.: Jalmar Press, 1971), are practical tools for introducing TA to children.
3 Claude Steiner, *Games Alcoholics Play* (New York: Grove Press, 1971).
4 Ibid., chap. 16.

Chapter 6

1 Stephen Karpman, "Fairy Tales and Script Drama Analysis," *Transactional Analysis Bulletin* 7 (April 1968).
2 Further injunction information is provided by Robert Goulding and Mary Goulding in their article "Injunctions, Decisions, and Redecisions," *Transactional Analysis Journal* (January 1976), and in "New Directions in Transactional Analysis. Creating an Environment for Redecision and Change," in C. Sager and H. Kaplan, *Progress in Group and Family Therapy* (New York: Brunner-Mazel, 1972).
3 Thomas A. Harris, *I'm O.K.—You're O.K.* (New York: Harper & Row, 1969), provides a comprehensive description of the four life positions.
4 Eric Berne, *What Do You Say After You Say Hello?* (New York: Grove Press, 1972), chap. 8.
5 Ibid.

Chapter 7

1 Eric Berne, *Games People Play* (New York: Grove Press, 1964),

provides a detailed description of life, marital, party, sexual, underworld, consulting-room and good games. Berne's work is the basis for the applications to fat fever.

Chapter 8

1 Eric Berne, *What Do You Say After You Say Hello?* (New York: Grove Press, 1972), chap. 2.

Chapter 9

1 Persons interested in in-depth reparenting will benefit from Jacqui Schiff's (with Beth Day) *All My Children* (New York: M. Evans, 1970) and *The Cathexis Reader* by the Cathexis Institute Staff and others, 1975.
2 Spot reparenting refers to identifying specific issues, cathecting young to the source incidents, and replacing the destructive or uncomfortable Parent messages which energize the issue. For further information, see Russel Osnes, "Spot Reparenting," *Transactional Analysis Journal* (July 1974).
3 Self-reparenting is a technique for self-restructuring of the Parent. Muriel James, "Self-Reparenting Theory and Process," *Transactional Analysis Journal* (July 1974), provides an effective description of the theory and process.
4 Eric Berne, *What Do You Say After You Say Hello?* (New York: Grove Press, 1972), chap. 9.
5 Robert and Mary Goulding refer to this approach as Gestalt dream work in "Injunctions, Decisions, and Redecisions," *Transactional Analysis Journal* (January 1975).
6 Sigmund Freud, *The Interpretation of Dreams* (New York: Basic Books, 1955).
7 T.M. French and E. Fromm, *Dream Interpretation* (New York: Basic Books, 1964).

Chapter 10

1 The International Transactional Analysis Association maintains a list of qualified therapists. Write ITAA, 1772 Vallejo Street, San Francisco, California 94123
2 Those persons who would like more detailed information on life scripts are directed to:

- Paul MacCormick, "Guide for Use of a Life Script in Transactional Analysis," which provides a questionnaire and example interviews.
- Eric Berne, *What Do You Say After You Say Hello?* (New York: Grove Press, 1972), chap. 23, provides a comprehensive script checklist covering prenatal influences, early, middle, and later childhood, adolescence, maturity, death, biological factors, choice of therapists, script signs, treatment, and therapy plus a condensed script analysis checklist.
- Claude Steiner, *Scripts People Live: Transactional Analysis of Life Scripts* (New York: Grove Press, 1974), describes clearly life plans and the use of TA in changing life plans or scripts.

3 Muriel James, "Self-Reparenting Theory and Process," *Transactional Analysis Journal* (July 1974).

4 TA's three "P's" are Potency, Permission, and Protection. Patricia Crossman, "Permission and Protection," *Transactional Analysis Bulletin,* 8 (July 1969). Eric Berne, *What Do You Say After You Say Hello?* chap. 19, describes the application of the three "P's" in therapy.

5 Muriel James, *What Do You Do with Them Now That You've Got Them?* (Reading, Mass.: Addison-Wesley, 1974).

Chapter 11

1 Edgar A. Guest, "It Couldn't Be Done," in *The Path to Home* (Chicago: Reilly Lee, 1919).

GLOSSARY

Activities The useful projects or tasks which are productive for ourselves and others.

Adapted Child The subpersonality of the Child ego state which complies, accepts, and follows.

Adult The nonfeeling ego state which is the rational, logical part of each individual.

Bathroom A family pattern which is bowel-oriented.

Child The ego state which contains the feelings and adaptations experienced in childhood.

Cold Stroke A unit of recognition which stimulates bad feelings.

Commitment A personal decision to follow a course of action toward a permanent cure.

Condition Category Categorizing people by comparing their actual weight to the appropriate healthy weight for their sex, height, and body structure.

Contamination A condition which occurs when the Adult accepts Parent or Child inputs as factual data.

Contract An explicit agreement which establishes cure activities and goals.

Controlling Parent The subpersonality of the Parent ego state which judges, controls, and criticizes.

Critical Condition A person more than 25 pounds over his or her appropriate weight.

Discount An action which reduces the value of a stroke or the feeling of worth of an individual.

Drama A real-life drama in which participants assume Persecutor, Victim, and Rescuer roles in a Drama Triangle. During the Drama, the roles switch, resulting in unexpected action, response, or outcome, much as in a fine play.

Ego State The feelings and experiences in each individual which stimulate a consistent pattern of behavior.

Family Pattern An orientation adopted by a family which establishes their standards and norms and which continues to influence lifelong feelings and behavior.

Free Child The subpersonality of the Child ego state which is hedonistic, unfettered, and fun-loving.

Gallows Transaction The inappropriate signs, words, gestures, and laughs which reinforce destructive or tragic behavior.

Game A life Drama in which the transactions appear plausible but contain an ulterior motive. The game ends with one or more players being hurt physically or emotionally.

Helping Parent The subpersonality of the Parent ego state which nurtures and helps.

Hidden Transactions Communications which appear plausible on one level but contain a hidden psychological message or motive.

Hurt A family pattern which is hostility-oriented.

Injunction The "Don't" messages or commands programmed or accepted in childhood which continue to restrain a person from feeling, thinking, and acting for herself or himself.

Intimacy An honest relationship with spontaneous expressions of love, caring, empathy, and appreciation. Intimacy is devoid of crooked or ritualistic games or rackets.

Kitchen A family pattern which is food- and Kitchen-oriented.

Life Positions Positions of O.K.-ness and not-O.K.-ness which individuals adopt and which describe how they feel about themselves and others.

Life Script A life plan based on childhood decisions which commit an individual to an ongoing pattern of behavior. The decisions are reinforced by events and parents and form the basis of the individual's character.

Little Professor The subpersonality of the Child ego state which contains intuitive, creative, manipulative, unschooled wisdom.

Loser A person who fails to reach his or her goals. Persons who follow destructive patterns blindly are losers.

Love A family pattern which is empathy-, caring-, sharing-, and affection-oriented.

Mild Condition A person 6 to 12 pounds over his or her appropriate weight.

No Surprise Transaction A communication which gets an expected response.

Parent The ego state which contains the feelings, attitudes, and behaviors modeled after significant parental figures.

Pastimes The harmless conversations which require very little real involvement and commitment from participants.

Patience The characteristic which enables a person to move slowly and surely toward a permanent change.

Pattern A life style initiated by parental messages and example.

Permission An Adult intervention which allows a person to disobey the parental tapes.

Persecutor The power and influence Drama role from which force is applied.

Potency The understanding and knowledge which provide an individual with the power and capability to initiate a change.

Protection The Adult input which establishes that it is safe to disobey parental injunctions.

Racket A recurring feeling which a person regularly displays.

Redecision The change of feelings and behaviors which amends a family pattern and life plan.

Reparent The action which replaces harmful parental messages with more appropriate, comfortable, healthy messages.

Rescuer The Drama role assumed by the Parent or Child savior.

Ritual Recurring events which follow a set pattern.

Serious Condition A person 13 to 25 pounds over his or her appropriate weight.

Stamps A person's collection of good and bad feelings which are traded as Permission for some action or payoff.

Stroke A unit of recognition.

Stroking The act of recognizing.

Surprise Transaction A communication which gets an unexpected response.

Transactional Analysis (TA) A model for understanding human behavior and for analyzing our various selves, the transactions between people, and our life positions. TA emphasizes that we have control of ourselves and that we can change ourselves if we so desire.

Transactions The verbal or nonverbal communications and interactions between two or more persons.

Victim The Drama role which is the object of force and power.

Warm Stroke A unit of recognition which stimulates good feelings.

Warning Condition A person 4 to 6 pounds over his or her appropriate weight.

Winner A person who reaches his or her objectives. Persons who make the pattern changes necessary for successful goal completion are winners.

Withdrawal The act of physically or mentally removing oneself from involvement with others.

Zigzag Stroke A unit of recognition which appears warm but contains a cold, hidden condition.

BIBLIOGRAPHY

Berne, Eric. *Transactional Analysis in Psychotherapy*. New York: Grove Press, 1961.

———. *Games People Play*. New York: Grove Press, 1964.

———. *What Do You Say After You Say Hello?* New York: Grove Press, 1972.

Cathexis Institute Staff and others. *Cathexis Reader*. 1975.

Foulkes, David. *The Psychology of Sleep*. New York: Scribner's, 1966.

Freed, Alvyn. *TA For Kids*. Sacramento, Calif.: Jalmar Press, 1971.

———. *TA For Tots*. Sacramento, Calif.: Jalmar Press, 1973.

Freud, Sigmund. *The Interpretation of Dreams*. New York: Basic Books, 1955.

Fromm, E. and French, T.M. *Dream Interpretation*. New York: Basic Books, 1964.

Harris, Thomas A. *I'm OK—You're OK*. New York: Harper & Row, 1967.

James, Muriel and Jongeward, Dorothy. *Born To Win*. Reading, Mass.: Addison-Wesley, 1971.

James, Muriel. *What Do You Do with Them Now That You've Got Them?* Reading, Mass.: Addison-Wesley, 1974.

Jongeward, Dorothy and Scott, Dru. *Women As Winners*. Reading, Mass.: Addison-Wesley, 1976.

Schiff, Jacqui with Day, Beth. *All My Children*. New York: M. Evans, 1970.

Steiner, Claude. *Games Alcoholics Play*. New York: Grove Press, 1971.

———. *Scripts People Live*. New York: Grove Press, 1974.

INDEX